Men Bleed Too

Men Bleed Too

✦

A Compelling Story About One Man's Struggle to Help His Wife Fight Breast Cancer!

Thomas Brown

iUniverse, Inc.

New York Lincoln Shanghai

Men Bleed Too
A Compelling Story About One Man's Struggle to Help His Wife Fight Breast Cancer!

Copyright © 2005 by Thomas E. Brown Jr.

iUniverse books may be ordered through booksellers or by contacting:

iUniverse
2021 Pine Lake Road, Suite 100
Lincoln, NE 68512
www.iuniverse.com
1-800-Authors (1-800-288-4677)

ISBN-13: 978-0-595-36187-8 (pbk)
ISBN-13: 978-0-595-67347-6 (cloth)
ISBN-13: 978-0-595-80634-8 (ebk)
ISBN-10: 0-595-36187-0 (pbk)
ISBN-10: 0-595-67347-3 (cloth)
ISBN-10: 0-595-80634-1 (ebk)

Printed in the United States of America

Contents

Acknowledgments

To all the women of the world that have dealt with breast cancer, I offer you my support for victory. May your inner strength and courage see you through this crisis. To Mary Ann Keller, a nurse and breast cancer survivor, thank you for taking the time to be the first reader of my rough draft. Your constructive criticism helped make this final product possible. I also owe a great deal of thanks to Rebecca Pratt of the Pratt Literary Agency. Thank you for all your help, suggestions, and patience. To my dear wife, Connie, who pushed me to tell this story, I thank you with all my heart. You were always there for me when I needed your strength and encouragement.

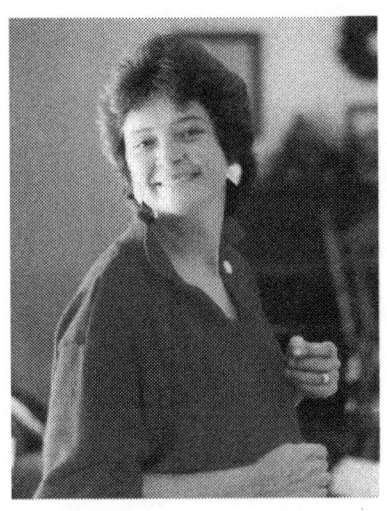

BARBARA

As I lay beside her, I felt
The warmth of her body
Exuding a physical presence
That stirred a memory of
A forgotten emotion. Until
I realized that it wasn't
The physical warmth that
I felt. It was in fact a
Deeper warmth of human kindness
That she gives so freely to
All she meets, and it embraces
Them in her genuine love
And concern.

> Thomas E. Brown Jr.
> March 2, 1985
> Osnabruck, Germany

PROLOGUE

This is a story about my first wife, Barbara, and her fight with breast cancer. We received the news in December 1992 that the tumor in Barbara's right breast was cancerous. It was classified as inflammatory breast cancer. This type of cancer is only one of the many forms of breast cancer, but the most dangerous. At the time we were both forty-four years old. I was a colonel in the U.S. Army serving as an instructor at the Command and General Staff College in Fort Leavenworth, Kansas, which is in northeast Kansas. Barbara was a housewife and the mother of our two sons, Thomas Robert and Jason Michael. Both of the boys were students at the University of Kansas, in Lawrence, about fifty miles to the southwest. Leavenworth was also my hometown. As such my parents, two brothers, and two sisters all lived in or around the Kansas City metro area.

When we received the confirmation that the extraction from a recent biopsy was indeed cancerous, I had a poor understanding of cancer, let alone this particular form that seemed to strike only females. I had no idea how prevalent the disease was among American women. However, with a little research I was quick to learn that in the United States, one in every nine women in their lifetime would develop breast cancer. I was shocked at the high statistics and decided that I needed to educate myself about the disease and the kinds of treatment options that were available. I searched the libraries and found several books written by women about their own experiences and the experiences of other women, but I found nothing written by a man. It was then that I thought I should start keeping a daily journal that I might one day turn into a book to help other men facing the same challenge.

The journal became my focal point for each day. I chronicled all the events from December 1992 until Barbara's death in August 1994. During the almost two years we spent battling her cancer; I found that the journal became very important for a couple reasons. First, it contained all the information about the times, types, and amounts of drugs that Barbara had taken. This was helpful to attending doctors because Barbara had several bouts with infections that landed her in the hospital. With the information at hand, I could easily tell the doctors what they needed to know. Secondly, the journal provided me with a place to write out my thoughts and emotions. At the time, I looked at it as a routine just to keep track of events, but in retrospect, I find that it was a way for me to release pent-up pressure.

The National Breast Cancer Foundation predicts that in 2005, more than 211,000 women in the United States will be diagnosed with breast cancer, and 43,300 of them will die from the disease. Whether or not you or a loved one has been diagnosed with cancer, I believe that the information I provide in this book may help. My experience is only one of millions about fighting cancer. However, it will not be the last. It is my intent and hope that the thoughts and experiences that I share with you in this book will ease your burden.

In the chapters that follow, you will see the role that I played during our fight with cancer. I became the task manager and primary caregiver. I made all decisions concerning the treatment of the disease. It is a sad story, because Barbara ultimately died from cancer. However, it is a story rich in emotion, love, and logic that also details how this disease affected and changed our daily lives. If the information in this book helps someone who has a loved one battling cancer, then I will have accomplished my goal.

1

THE BEGINNINGS

December 10, 1992, in Leavenworth, Kansas was just as dreary as any other day in a midwestern winter. The sky was overcast, and there was a slight mist that wasn't snow but wasn't rain either. A damp chill permeated the air. At about 10:00 AM, I received the confirmation call about my wife's biopsy results. The call came from Major Richard Combs, M.D. The pathology report from a specimen taken from Barbara's right breast was cancerous.

Dr. Combs and I had a short conversation about the impact of the findings and set up an appointment for Barbara and me to go in and discuss the next step. Shock and despair mixed together to envelop me in a cocoon of self-pity at that moment. Although I was thrown into a serious situation, totally void of background knowledge on how to deal with it, I decided to develop a strategy to best deal with what I had just been handed.

It was truly a sad day in our lives. Both of our lives had been filled with love and riches over many years of marriage. But the choices for dealing with breast cancer are sadly simple: either you go through treatment or risk certain death. That night, Barbara and I courageously came to the agreement that we were going to beat breast cancer with joint and aggressive action. I think that it was a remarkable gesture on her part. I mean think of it—she was just told that she had cancer. Yes, she was depressed—crying, asking, "Why me?" and responding in all the other ways that you would expect. But she had enough character and presence of mind to agree to an aggressive scheme to go after and defeat the cancer. I tell you this now because it is the single driving force that kept her going through a tremendous amount of pain and depression for almost two years. So, where did all that character come from? And how was she able to muster so much courage at the very beginning when her mind reeled at the thought of dying at forty-four?

Barbara was truly a remarkable woman. I had known her since she was sixteen years old, and I was married to her for twenty-five-and-half years. In all that time, I can't think of a single person who met Barbara who didn't instantly feel her genuine warmth. She always had a kind word to offer along with an infectious laugh and a beautiful smile.

She was born October 21, 1948, in Mineola, New York, to Robert A. Domos, the son of a Hungarian immigrant, and Evva Marie Brieson, the daughter of a Cherokee Indian. Barbara was the second child of the marriage. At the time of her birth, she had a sister, Susan, who was three. The young Domos family was an Army family. Robert, who served in the World War II, was soon promoted to the rank of captain and shortly received orders to move to Heidelberg, Germany. Tragically, while stationed in Germany, Evva died. Barbara had been about five years old then and, later, had faint memories about her mother, but she did speak fondly about Evva's mother, Grandma Brieson, who stayed with the girls and helped the grieving family.

Robert moved on with his life. Caring for two young girls and maintaining a profession as an Army officer was a difficult task at best. In 1954, he met and married Catherine Aileen O'Toole. They moved to an obscure Army post in the deep woods of Missouri called Fort Leonard Wood, which was named after a famous Civil War general. It was here in 1955 that the first of two brothers, Robert Jr., was born to the newly formed Domos family. Brother John eventually joined the family in 1958.

By now, Robert Sr. had attained the rank of major and was moved on to a posting in Taiwan in 1959. Barbara's accounts of her time in Taiwan reflected good memories. The younger brothers rapidly learned to speak Chinese, and life in the Department of Defense elementary schools was pretty good overall. The stay in the Far East ended in 1961 when the family moved to Fort Leavenworth, Kansas.

Barbara entered the Catholic school system at St. Joseph in Leavenworth in sixth grade. After graduating from eighth grade, she moved on to the Catholic high school, Immaculata. She went through the typical awkward stage that girls do in their first year of high school—braces on her teeth, skinny, and not fully developed. But by the fall of her sophomore year, she had developed into a beautiful young lady.

My fascination with her began during the fall of 1964. I remember our first encounter at a football game. I was a shy high school junior and wanted to meet her; she was a sophomore cheerleader who was beautiful and didn't know that I existed. I finally got up enough courage to go up to her at half time and introduce myself. It was an awkward moment for me, but Barbara was very nice, and soon after, we had our first date. After a month of dating, we decided to go steady. We dated throughout the remainder of that year.

The bad news of her father's transfer came in the spring of 1965. He was reassigned as a special services officer to Okinawa, Japan. The plan was for him to go ahead of the family and establish a place to live while the children finished the school year in Leavenworth.

Barbara and I spent a lot of time together during the rest of my junior year. The summer came and went too quickly. We were eventually faced with the fact that she was going to leave soon and that we wouldn't see each other for at least a year. We were young and in love. We vowed to each other that after Barbara graduated from high school, she would return to Leavenworth. We agreed that we would each date other people but retain our true love for each other.

The fall rolled around, and we started back to school. Soon the word came that her father had found a set of Army quarters, and her mother Aileen began to make preparations for the move to Okinawa.

Barbara, her mother, and her two brothers flew out of the Kansas City airport on November 11, 1965. Barbara's sister, Sue, stayed in Leavenworth and enrolled as a freshman at Saint Mary College. It was a day that truly broke my heart. I was seventeen, deeply in love, and faced with the reality that I might not ever see the girl of my dreams again. During our final days together, I made her promise no matter what happened in our lives, she would at least give me a call when she returned to the United States—if for no other reason, just to let me know that she was all right. I finished my senior year, graduated, and went off to college. During this time, Barbara and I wrote each other often. At first, it seemed as though everything would work out as we had planned. Then at the end of her senior year, in May 1967, her father informed her that his term had been extended for another year and that she had to remain with the family. We continued to write for a year, but things soon faded, and the once-cherished love affair ended—or at least that's how it seemed at the time.

In June 1968, I received that promised call from Barbara who was now back in the United States staying with relatives in Phoenix, Arizona. Barbara told me that she would very much like to see me again. We phoned back and forth for about a month, and then she decided to move back to Leavenworth. Barbara moved into an apartment with her best friend, Peggy Jackson, and went to work for Hallmark Cards. It did not take us long to rekindle our love for each other. We continued to date throughout the summer, and in September I returned to college at the University of Kansas in Lawrence. Barbara stayed in Leavenworth, but we saw each other about every weekend. By late fall we realized that marriage was the next step and became engaged. We planned a spring wedding in 1969 to coincide with her parents' return to the United States. However, we were both so eager to get married that we changed the date to December 28, 1968. I was in my junior year of college at the time. I finished college in June 1970 and received a commission as a second lieutenant in the U.S. Army. Our oldest son, Thomas Robert, was born on July 1, 1970, and shortly afterward we set off for our first assignment in Fort Knox, Kentucky. After a series of assignments, our second son, Jason Michael, was born on October 25, 1973, in Nuremberg, Germany.

Our Army life was filled with exciting and challenging assignments. Over the years we developed many friends that eventually became a vital support group for Barbara during her fight with cancer. For over twenty-five-and-a-half years Barbara followed me around the world with the Army, raised two children, and provided me with invaluable counsel. She was truly a wonderful mother, my partner in marriage, and my best friend.

Barbara's strong will and character were evident from the beginning. Her father recounts that when she was a little girl, she was the one with the skinned knees. She was a fighter and a provider. She was honest, kind, and thoughtful, and she always cared for others. She had the type of personality that lights up a room. She made and retained friends quickly. She was a decent Christian and, until November 1992, was in perfect health.

2

DISCOVERY AND INITIAL TREATMENT

Barbara first noticed that something was unusual with her right breast in early November 1992. She always conducted monthly breast exams, but this month redness appeared. Her initial thoughts were that it was something to do with her menstrual cycle; she always had swelling of the breasts with her period. However, when the redness persisted, she became a bit more concerned. With more self-exams, she came to the conclusion that this was something out of the ordinary.

The holiday season was rapidly approaching, and we were having my family over for Thanksgiving dinner. About a week before Thanksgiving, Barbara told me for the first time that she suspected something unusual. She showed me the redness and asked me to feel around to see if I could detect a lump. The redness was very light and ran in a streak about a quarter of an inch wide along the breast from the armpit to the nipple. I felt the area up around the arm just below the shoulder. To me it felt like a very developed pectoral muscle. There was no indication of a lump or nodule at all. I felt the other breast in the same general area to make a comparison. They both felt generally the same. We discussed it and decided to wait until after she completed her period to see if the redness cleared up any. She did promise to make an appointment to see a doctor just to be sure. Up until this point, Barbara had never had a mammogram.

Thanksgiving came and went, her period ended, but the redness on her breast did not. She made an appointment to see a doctor for the third of December. I took her to the hospital, checked in, and sat with her in the waiting room. When the nurse called out her name, I gave her a hug, offered what I could for encouragement, and asked whether she wanted me to go with her. She told me that she would go alone. The exam yielded the same conclusion that Barbara and I had come to in November: something was unusual because of the redness, but the doctor felt no discernible lump.

I joined Barbara for a discussion with the doctor after the exam. He said that he wanted to get a mammogram conducted just to be positive. The military hospital only had one mammogram machine and technician. The doctor said that there could be a delay of up to two weeks to get on the schedule, so our choices were to wait or to contact a civilian hospital for something quicker. He wrote out a referral, and we went down to the clinic to make an appointment. As luck came our way, the technician had a cancellation and was free to conduct Barbara's mammogram immediately.

I went into the exam room and tried to provide comfort for Barbara, who was very scared by now. I helped her disrobe and put on the exam gown but had to leave the room during the actual exam. At the conclusion, the technician came out and told me that I could return to the exam room. I asked Barbara how it went, and her general reply was "OK." She described the procedure to me and showed me the various positions that she had to get in for the exam. Basically, the machine looks like some kind of a press. There is a platform where the patient places her breast, and then the top part moves down and smashes the breast like a pancake. Barbara said that it didn't hurt, but it was uncomfortable.

That night Dr. Combs called Barbara and said that he wanted to see us both the next day to discuss the results of the mammogram. We went back to the hospital on December 4. He showed us the mammogram picture and said it looked "suspicious." He told Barbara that he wanted to schedule her for a biopsy. We both looked at each other and tried to figure out what "suspicious" meant. I think at that point we mentally came to the same conclusion, but still hoped for the best.

I didn't know a lot about the internal anatomy of a female. I also did not know that women routinely have lumps in their breasts that are never cancerous. All I could think of was that the news was not good. The doctor at this point was noncommittal. I think that this was probably a good thing. As a surgeon and a problem solver, he did not have all the facts necessary to make a diagnosis. He simply was following a routine that many hours of study in medical school and practical experience directed him toward. It was certainly not the time to discuss gloom and doom, nor would it have been appropriate to provide false hope. I've often wondered what kind of training doctors receive that helps them deal with giving people bad news. It must be an emotional strain on them, too, even though they are looking primarily at the clinical side of things. At any rate, Dr. Combs was very kind and considerate and answered our questions.

Dr. Combs told Barb that he had scheduled her for a biopsy on Monday, December 7, and that she needed to go to the lab for blood work and preoperative checks. So for the next couple of hours, we wandered from clinic to clinic processing the forms that we received at the admissions desk. By the time we left the hospital, we were both scared. Barbara couldn't stop crying. I tried to console her, but it just didn't seem to help. When we got home, I told her that getting all upset would not help the situation. We both agreed that we would have to take this one step at a time. I knew that the strength to fight was hidden deep inside my wife, but that I would have to be the one to push her along and provide constant encouragement. We also decided not to say anything to our sons at that time because we didn't know if we were dealing with cancer or just a benign lump.

After supper that night, I went downstairs and sat on the couch. Barb was in our bedroom upstairs. I knew that we each needed some privacy and time alone. I had a rotten feeling in my gut, and I was overcome with emotion. I began to cry. I was depressed at the thought that my wife might have to go through a battle with cancer. I felt anger and resentment. I kept telling myself that we did not deserve such a turn of events.

Barbara and I decided not to tell a lot of people about her possible condition. Of course, we both hoped and prayed that it would turn out well. I did tell my parents, who also lived in Leavenworth. My mother talked to one of my cousins, Sharon Concannon, who had had several lumps removed from her breasts the previous few years. Sharon called Barbara that weekend and explained, step-by-step, each procedure the doctors would take during the biopsy. I think this made Barbara somewhat more relaxed since she now had more knowledge about the procedure. I think it was also consoling for her to hear it from another woman and a relative.

Monday morning arrived a lot sooner than either of us wanted. We checked into the hospital around 6:30 AM. I helped Barb get into her hospital gown, and then I took her clothing to her recovery room. I went back waited with Barbara for the surgical nurse to arrive. She came around 7:30, put a surgical cap on Barb's head, and told her it was time to go into surgery. I gave Barb a kiss and a hug, told her not to worry, and reminded her that I would see her in the recovery room.

The waiting area outside the surgical clinic at Munson Army Health Center in Fort Leavenworth consisted of a row of fixed chairs along a wall. I found a magazine and a cup of coffee and sat down. People of all sorts passed through the area; most were quiet for their own reasons. It seemed like the operation was taking quite a long time, but I guess that I was just nervous.

At around 9:00, Dr. Combs came into the waiting area. I stood up and asked him how the operation went. He said that the surgery went well and that Barbara was fine but still under the influence of the anesthesia. When I asked him what was next, he suggested that we go into a private room to talk. We went into a small TV room just off the hallway. During our conversation, I asked him to explain the procedures that he used to perform the biopsy. He said that he removed a piece of the tumor about the size of a quarter and that the sample would have to be sent to a pathology lab for complete analysis. I asked him what it looked like, and he responded that it looked like a malignant tumor. In fact, he added that if the pathology report came back negative, he would order another biopsy. I got a huge knot in my stomach. I tried to remain logical and unemotional. I knew that Barbara would be devastated by the news so I decided not to tell her, but just to wait for the official report.

Barb came out of the recovery room a little groggy but ready to get out of the hospital. After she proved to the head nurse that she could eat without getting sick and urinate, she was released. On the way home she questioned me about my conversation with the surgeon, but I didn't tell her the whole story. When we got home, Barb was exhausted. She rested for the remainder of the day. I left her alone and escaped to the seclusion of the downstairs sofa, suffering severe depression and anxiety over the suspicions that the doctor and I shared.

The next night as Barb and I talked in bed, I couldn't keep it from her anymore. Slowly, and as easily as I could, I told her the rest of the story about my conversation with Dr. Combs. To my surprise, her only response was that she already knew that the tumor was cancerous. I asked her how she knew, and she told me that it was just a feeling. We hugged, had a good cry together, and went to sleep.

After I arrived home from work the next evening, Barbara and I agreed that we needed to tell our sons. We did not have all the information concerning treatment, but we felt they needed to know she had cancer. I talked to both of them that evening and we all agreed that their mother was a fighter. I told them that as soon as we had more information, I would give them a call.

The next trip back to the hospital was on December 15. During our visit with Dr. Combs we had a thousand questions. He answered them as we went along. We discussed the various options available and collectively agreed that Barb would see an oncologist in Kansas City at the Cancer Center of the University of Kansas Medical Center. We drove to KU Medical Center the next day for our first appointment with Dr. Rene Ramos.

Upon arriving at the Cancer Center, we were directed to a waiting room. Soon a nurse appeared and asked us to go into one of the small exam rooms, where she told Barbara to disrobe from the waist up. The nurse then conducted the routine screening of blood pressure, temperature, and height and weight. In a short time Dr. Ramos arrived.

The doctor was a gentle man and had a pleasing personality that seemed to calm Barbara down a little. He went over Barbara's medical history by asking a series of questions. At one point he asked, "Are you a smoker?" to which Barb responded, "No, I quit last night." That in itself was a difficult feat because she had been smoking for over twenty years. The doctor looked up and said, "Well that doesn't matter anyway, because smoking has nothing to do with breast cancer."

At that point my beloved gave me the hardest stare of my life. I had always told her to quit, and when the determination of cancer came up, I told her that she had to quit so as not to exacerbate an already bad situation. The look that I got was one of disgust. So now it was my fault that she was having nicotine withdrawal. I must say, however, that she stuck to her vow and never smoked again.

Dr. Ramos conducted a thorough exam and then explained the course of action that he felt best-suited Barb's needs. We asked about the chances of recovery and the possibility of recurrence. He told us that because Barbara had inflammatory breast cancer that the chances of recurrence after treatment were about 60 percent. However, if she made it past five years, then her chances of long-term survival increased to about 80 percent. It was not pleasant news, but at least he was honest with us and did provide some hope for a cure.

Dr. Ramos went on to explain that he wanted Barb to start off with a bone scan and a CAT scan to establish a baseline of her physical condition, and that he wanted to start chemotherapy immediately. He felt that the tumor was too large at this point for Barbara to have a mastectomy and that the chances of it spreading to other parts of the body were very high. The schedule that he prescribed was four months of chemotherapy to shrink and contain the mass, followed by a modified radical mastectomy. After the operation, Barbara would receive additional chemotherapy, which he termed "adjunct treatment" to kill off any remaining microscopic cancer cells that might be lingering in her system.

After our discussion with the doctor, he left the exam room, and Barb put her clothes back on. I could tell that she was very upset, but she was hanging in there just the same. I tried to console her and reassure her that our commitment together to fight this thing with all our strength would get us through this difficult period. She acknowledged my support. We left the exam room and went out to meet with Dr. Ramos's nurse who briefed us on what to expect from the chemotherapy. Nurse Barbara Jordan, L.P.N., was gentle but frank with us. She gave us several brochures and pamphlets describing the effects of chemotherapy. She also went on to explain the cycle that the doctor had prescribed. In simplest terms it went like this: on day one Barb would receive chemotherapy by injection, and eight days later the same thing. In addition, she would take chemotherapy by pill for fourteen days, stop for a week to recover and allow the white blood cells time to build back up, and then start the cycle all over again. The nurse directed Barb to get weekly blood draws to monitor her red and white cell count. Barb was very upset and couldn't stop crying. Both the nurse and I tried to console her, but she just responded by saying that she would be all right—that she was just a very emotional person.

Before we left the doctor's office, we made an appointment for December 17 for the first chemotherapy treatment. We proceeded to the third floor of the hospital and checked in to the radiology clinic. The bone scan and CAT scan were pretty uneventful except for the quart of barium that Barbara had to drink and the radioisotope injection, which left a very nasty bruise on her arm. On the way home, we stopped and picked up some supper. It had been a very long and strenuous day.

The next morning Barbara informed me that her menstrual cycle had begun. I note that because this would be the next to the last period that she would ever have. The effects of the chemotherapy would very quickly kick her into menopause at forty-four years of age.

On December 17, we arrived at the KU Cancer Center on time and were greeted by a friendly staff. After the front-desk staff performed the usual new-patient procedures of insurance information and opening a file, Barbara and I were escorted to the treatment facility. Nurse Mary Murphy, L.P.N., put a small needle in Barbara's arm and started injecting dextrose followed by dexamethasone and ondansetron. The dextrose was used as a flush, while the other two were to help ward off nausea. Nurse Mary then came back with the chemotherapy drugs. She had two vials of Adriamycin (which is yellow) and one vial of fluorouracil, or 5FU, (which is red). She attached a needle to the first vial, placed it in the butterfly port and "pushed" the drug into Barb's vein. The whole procedure took about an hour.

On the way out, we went to the Cancer Center pharmacy and were briefed on the additional drugs that Barb had to take. She was given another cancer drug called Cytoxan. The pharmacist explained that Barb was to take the Cytoxan three times a day for fourteen days. Barb also received diphenhydramine and

Compazine. These pills were designed to help ward off the nausea that would be produced by the Cytoxan. She was to take each pill twice a day or more if she was really feeling sick to her stomach.

We grabbed our bag of drugs, wrote down the next scheduled appointment, and left the hospital. I accompanied Barb to the restroom and noticed that her urine was very red; it wasn't blood, but residue of the 5FU. As we walked across the parking lot to our car, I noticed that Barb looked yellow but didn't say anything, thinking that it might just be the lighting in the parking lot. Later that night she asked me, "Do I look yellow?" and told me her lips felt a little numb.

3

CHEMOTHERAPY EFFECTS AND BATTLING INFECTIONS

The day after Barb's first chemotherapy treatment, she tried to go on with her life in the usual fashion. It was a cold bleary winter day but that didn't dampen her shopping spirits. Barb and my mom and dad had always gotten along very well. In fact she was more like an older daughter than a daughter-in-law. So, on the cold winter day of December 18, 1992, they set off for Kansas City and the shopping malls. When she got home that night I noticed that her cheeks looked a little red, and there was redness above her right eye. I figured that it was just from being out in the cold, but several hours later it was still there. That night as we prepared for bed I looked at her right breast where the tumor was located. It, too, was red and angry looking.

The next few days, Barb was nauseous and tired. She stayed in bed most of the day and often complained that the tumor was really beginning to become uncomfortable. We tried to make light of the situation by saying that the chemotherapy was doing its stuff and killing off the nasty, old tumor. Barb told me that she was constipated but her appetite remained pretty good.

By December 21, Barb was drained of energy. She was nauseated most of the time and began coughing a lot and spitting up a lot of phlegm. At that point we couldn't figure out whether it was caused by the chemotherapy or because she had just quit smoking, and her lungs were trying to clear up.

Two days later, the first bout of vomiting occurred. She told me that she ate some toast for breakfast and a sandwich for lunch and had taken her pills to ward off the sickness. I managed to get her to get out of bed and to go for a short walk. When we came back around 5:45 PM, the vomiting began again. It was short but violent. Within the next hour she threw up about four more times. I tried to help as much as I could, but there was nothing I could do other than clean up the mess. Before she went to sleep she complained that her stomach muscles were sore. We concluded that it was from all the throwing up.

The next day was Christmas Eve. I can still see her standing in front of our Christmas tree, and my only thought at the time was: "Will she still be alive next year at this time?" I was really having a rough time seeing her so sick. I literally hated the idea of the chemotherapy drugs being pumped into her veins to kill off cancer cells. It was sad and barbaric, but I soon came to realize that the definition of modern medicine in the treatment of cancer came down to very few options—radiation, surgery, and chemotherapy. It was truly depressing to watch a beautiful young woman being destroyed by the drugs that were supposed to help save her life. Even sadder was that we had only two options: take the treatment and hope for the best or watch the cancer cells spread throughout her body and eventually kill her.

Christmas Eve day saw us back at the Cancer Center for the second round of injected chemotherapy. We went back to Leavenworth that night, spent some time with family and friends. Barb said that she felt pretty good. I think a lot of it was getting out of the house and spending time with our sons and the rest of my family. Her menstrual cycle continued with a heavy blood flow and a lot of cramps. This didn't help her feel any better.

On Christmas morning we exchanged gifts with our sons and each other. Barbara told me that she really felt pretty good. That afternoon we went to my parent's house. There was plenty of food and drink and everyone had a wonderful time. It was a very good day for all of us, being around family and friends. I think it helped lift Barbara's spirits.

The next few days Barb was pretty tired and didn't have a lot of energy. She complained about being lightheaded and dizzy. She spent most of the time in bed. I kept her water glass filled with cold fluids and ice. I also tried to make sure that she ate something healthy even though her appetite was not the best in the world. She fluctuated between being constipated and having diarrhea. Her menstrual cycle was starting to come to an end.

December 28, 1992, and our twenty-fourth anniversary arrived. It had always been a joyous occasion. It was still joyous, but that year we found that the part of our vows that talked of sickness and health were coming all too true. We were both thankful of the life that we had together. We had two wonderful sons, great families, and, other than Barbara's tubal ligation and the delivery of two baby boys, neither of us had spent a day in the hospital. We had a perfect relationship filled with trust and compassion. We complemented each other and had a great ability to communicate and share our ideas. But this anniversary was different.

We still rejoiced but were so overcome with dealing with the problems of cancer that the day seemed routine.

The next morning, I fixed a pot of coffee, and Barb got out of bed to join me. She hadn't had a cup for several weeks because, besides destroying body cells, the chemotherapy also took away her taste buds. Most everything tasted like metal. But in her genuine spirit of love and concern for others, she pushed herself through all of this and sat down and had a cup of coffee with me. We went out that night to Father Charlie McGlinn's in Kansas City. My sister Linda was married to Pat McGlinn, and Father Charlie was his older brother. We always called him the family priest. We had a shrimp dinner and then left around 9:00 PM because I could tell that Barb was getting tired. Barbara's problem with constipation continued, and we decided it was time for a laxative to help relieve some of the pressure. By now, her lower gums were swollen and pinkish red.

On December 30, Barb finished taking the last of the Cytoxan pills for the first cycle of chemotherapy. She was really tired and not feeling well. Around 2:00 PM she had another violent vomiting session. She took some more diphenhydramine and Compazine after she threw up, and it seemed to help settle her stomach.

New Year's Eve found us at the Army hospital at 10:00 AM getting a blood draw. We had set up a schedule that allowed the medics at the Army hospital to draw and analyze the blood and then fax it to the Cancer Center in Kansas City. This saved us both time and money. The weekly blood draws were necessary for the oncology staff to monitor Barbara's progress and to look for any signs of danger. Later that afternoon, Nurse Barbara called from the Cancer Center to see how Barb was doing. I told her that she was real tired and that she had a couple of spells of vomiting. Nurse Barbara said that the blood count, particularly the white cells looked a little low. She told me to monitor Barb's temperature and that if it rose to 101 degrees to call the Cancer Center for instructions.

At 2:00 PM I took Barb's temperature. It was 99.8 degrees. Throughout the rest of the day I kept a close watch over her, and she said that she felt OK. She did ask me to go get her a vegetable tray because her teeth were hurting, and she felt like she needed something to chew on. Later in the day we got dressed and went over to some friends' house for a quiet New Year's Eve. We left early and returned home before the New Year arrived. At 9:30 PM Barb's temperature had climbed to 100.8 degrees. We both noted that she also had noticeable hair loss throughout the day. This is something that we knew would occur, but it was the one thing that Barbara hated the most out of everything that she had to go through.

On New Year's Day I jumped out of bed early, gave Barb a soft kiss, and assured her that this was the beginning of our healing year. I served her breakfast in bed consisting of scrambled eggs, toast, apple slices, and tomato slices. At 8:30 AM her temperature was 100.6 degrees. Barb was feeling really down and dejected and sorry for herself. She had hoped that by completing all of the Cytoxan that she would be feeling better by now. We had a long and good heart-to-heart talk about the healing process and how important it was to keep a positive attitude. She assured me that she was all right, just a little down but she was really trying hard to lick the nasty disease of cancer.

At 1:45 PM her temperature had climbed to 101 degrees. I called the Cancer Center and spoke with Dr. James Henry, M.D. Dr. Henry was the duty doctor for the day. I provided him with all the details and asked him to coordinate with the Army hospital in Leavenworth so we wouldn't have to drive to Kansas City. He called back shortly and said that I needed to take Barbara to the emergency room at the Army hospital. He said that Barb probably had an infection and that she needed some antibiotics to help fight it off since her own immune system was incapable of doing it alone. We arrived at the hospital about a half hour later, and the attending physician had a vial of blood drawn for analysis. The lab report came back that Barb's white blood cell count was 600. The normal range for a woman is somewhere between 4,800 and 10,800. The nurses then drew an additional three vials of blood for culture tests to see if they could isolate the infection. They started an IV drip of dextrose and sodium chloride and added a general antibiotic of gentamicin. A chest X-ray and a physical exam by the on-call internal medicine doctor, Dr. Jane Collins, M.D. followed all this up. Barbara liked Dr. Collins a lot. She felt very comfortable with a woman doctor. The doctor explained to us both that what occurred was not uncommon for cancer patients. Chemotherapy destroys so many white cells that it takes bone marrow a long time to replace the lost ones. During that time, the patient is likely to get an infection either from some of their own internal bacteria or catch something from someone else. She explained that the increase in body temperature was a sign that an infection of some kind was present. Dr. Collins admitted Barb to the hospital for treatment and observation.

The first four days in the hospital really didn't go well. The doctor checked daily on Barb's progress, but her white count was not increasing very rapidly. I spent as much time by Barbara's bedside as I could, talking and comforting her. She was really tired and not feeling well. The food was not good and the nurses kept her up most of the night changing the antibiotic IVs every four to eight hours. Barbara's hair was really starting to fall out by now. It was really a mess because it fell everywhere in the hospital room. I tried to keep it cleaned up and off of her food and sleeping gown, but it was an almost impossible task. When Barbara took a shower one day, I noticed that the shower walls were covered with her hair. We both agreed that it would be better to cut it all off so we wouldn't have to constantly fight the mess.

On the fifth day, I stopped by the hospital on my way to work. Dr. Collins said that Barb's white count had risen to 1,300 and she decided to release her at 1:00 PM. I picked her up that afternoon, took her home, and told her that I would stay with her the rest of the afternoon just in case she needed anything. Barb took a nice warm bath and immediately went to sleep. I watched her as she rested. She was completely exhausted. Her hair had really started to fall out. I felt so sorry for my beautiful wife. Of all the people in the world, why on earth did she have to have cancer?

The next day January 6, we went back to the Cancer Center for the third cycle of chemotherapy. But the doctors said that her white blood cell count was still too low and they only conducted a physical exam and told us to wait another week before starting the chemotherapy again. Dr. Ramos wanted to know how we were both doing. Barb asked him about the horrible heartburn that she had been experiencing. He responded that it was normal and he would prescribe some Zantac to relieve it. He also recommended that Barb be given a new drug called Neupogen, starting on the tenth day of her third chemotherapy cycle. He told us that it would stimulate her bone marrow to produce white cells a lot quicker. When we got back home that evening, Barbara told me that she wanted me to cut off the rest of her hair.

The hair cutting incident was something that Barbara hated the most of all the things that she went through. She had beautiful hair and was proud of it. She just hated the idea of being bald. I tried to console her and I reminded her of how much of a mess it was with it constantly falling out on her clothes and food. She told me that she knew all of that and that although she didn't want to get rid of it, she knew it was necessary. At first I used scissors to take off the big chunks and then I used a set of hair clippers to trim it down. I tried to leave a little on the top so that she wasn't totally bald. When I finished, she looked like some poor victim of a concentration camp. So I told her to sit back down and I would cut it a little closer. The final product resembled something closer to a fuzzy Sinead O'Connor. Around the house, Barbara at first covered her head with a scarf. She wore a wig whenever she left the house. Eventually she became more comfortable without a scarf in the house. As time went along, she eventually lost the rest of the short hairs and became completely bald, including her eyelashes and eyebrows.

The week of January 7 was the break that Barb really needed. She was able to eat well and get up and get around. She did some shopping. We went out to a couple of dinners and generally just started feeling somewhat normal again. During that week we had a heavy wet snowstorm. I got out the snow shovel and went out in the evening after work and started to clear off the driveway. About fifteen minutes after I started Barbara appeared, dressed in her moon boots, coat and scarf with the hood pulled up and fastened. It was a sight I will never forget. There she was sick with cancer, just out of the hospital for an infection, but willing to help me clear the snow. I looked up and told her to go back inside. She insisted on staying and helping me out. After a couple scoops, she tired and said she would go back inside. This brave little action on her part once again demonstrated to me the tremendous character and fighting spirit of the woman that I loved.

The rest of January was pretty much a standard routine. Barbara continued on the chemotherapy and was now in the second cycle. Her general attitude remained positive and she showed no signs of any real discomfort except from all the bruises on her arm caused by all the blood draws. We tried to live a normal life while fighting cancer. Barbara remained brave and strong and I constantly reassured her about how proud I was of her.

Our fourth trip to the Cancer Center was January 11. Barbara's white cell count was high enough for the nurses to give her the third treatment of chemotherapy. After the treatment we left with another new drug. This was the Neupogen that Dr. Ramos wanted Barbara to take to help stimulate the bone marrow to produce white cells and hopefully keep hers from crashing so low again. Fortunately for us, our next-door neighbor was a registered nurse. She agreed to give Barbara the daily shot of one milliliter of Neupogen. Barbara had her first shot on January 20 around 4:00 PM. No more than a half hour later she had a reaction and a violent vomiting spell. Later, I went to McDonald's to pick up some supper and Barbara ate a double cheeseburger with large fries. At least her appetite remained healthy. We couldn't figure out why she threw up, but she said that she just felt lousy all day.

On January 24, during the night and in the early morning, Barbara complained about being cold. She would get up to go pee and come back to bed shaking. At 7:30 AM her temperature was 99 degrees. I got up around 8:00 AM and tried to get her to eat something but she refused. She really looked tired and worn out, so I decided to stay home from church and monitor her temperature. Around 10:00 her temperature had climbed to 100.2 degrees. I let her sleep for a while and went back to check on her around 11:30. By then her temperature had climbed to 102.2 degrees. I called the Cancer Center and spoke with Dr. Henry again. It seemed like that poor guy was always pulling weekend duty. He said that Barbara needed to go to the emergency room because she probably had another infection. I called the ER at the Army hospital and told them about Barbara's medical history. We arrived at the hospital around 12:15 PM. The duty doctor in the ER was a family practitioner, so he went through the routine with a lot of questions, checking her vital signs, and having blood drawn for analysis. He called the on-call internal medicine doctor to come in to the ER. We weren't lucky enough to get Dr. Collins, but we did get Dr. Pitt, another female. When Dr. Pitt arrived she continued the exam. Barbara's temperature remained high and the initial blood draw indicated that her white count was 300. This was not good news considering that the Neupogen was supposed to help her produce white cells at a faster rate. After all the discussions, blood draws, physical exam and a call to Dr. Ramos, Barbara was admitted to the hospital again. The ER attending nurses had a difficult time finding a vein in Barbara's arm from which to take additional vials of blood for the routine culture tests.

When we got to the hospital room, the nurses on the IV team had a difficult time finding a place to put the needle in for the necessary IV drips. Both arms were severely bruised from all of the needle sticks from the previous blood draws. Eventually the nurses were able to find a vein and Barbara was given gentamicin and Fortaz, two types of antibiotics.

Throughout the rest of the week it was a routine schedule for me. I would get up early, make a lunch, and stop by Barb's hospital room on the way to work. At lunchtime I would go back over to the hospital, eat my lunch with her, and return to work. In the evenings I would go home, change clothes, and then go back to the hospital. The nursing staff was pretty good and allowed me to remain at night as long as I wanted. I really didn't mind the routine and the busy sched-ule that I had to keep to take care of the house chores and keeping myself fed. I felt so sorry for Barbara because she hated being sick and stuck in the hospital. At times it was difficult to console her. I did everything that I could to try to keep her spirits up. She always received lots of phone calls, cards, and flowers. She told me that the long time lying in bed made her back and butt sore. To help relieve this, I gave her back massages and butt rubs almost daily. I also tried to keep her well-supplied with reading material and little treats like chewing gum, candy bars, and her favorite: black licorice.

The nursing staff were all pretty good and Barbara received good care and attention. She did, however, like to try to do things on her own. One afternoon while I was visiting her in the hospital, she told me that she wanted to take a shower and wash what was left of her hair. I told her that I would help her because she was still very weak. In the meantime, I saw Dr. Combs in the hall and I stopped to talk to him for a few minutes. When I returned to the room I heard the shower water running. When I looked in, Barbara was sitting in a fetal position in the corner of the shower, crying. She was just too weak to stand. I helped her up, dried her off, and helped her get back into bed. She made a promise to me at that point that she would always let me help her in the future.

By January 26, Barbara was starting to feel a lot better. The nurses used Tylenol to break the fever any time it shot up. Barbara's white blood cell count had only risen to 400. Dr. Collins, the attending physician, took her off the Fortaz and added Timentin. Barbara completed her menstrual cycle, which helped her overall mental and physical state.

The next day Dr. Collins stopped by Barbara's room around 7:30 AM. She told us that the urine sample taken the previous Sunday revealed a bladder infection. She went on to add that if Barbara's temperature remained OK for the rest of the day that she would release her on Thursday morning. She also directed the nursing staff to stop the antibiotic IVs and go to a pill form using ciprofloxacin.

Barbara's temperature did remain stable and Dr. Collins released her the following morning. Her white cell count had climbed to 2,800. Maybe the Neupogen was working after all. That night at home we both held each other and had a good cry. I think it was one that was needed and well deserved. We both vowed to continue to fight but it seemed that for every step we took forward, we fell three back.

4

ATTITUDES AND ACTIONS

FEAR AND CONFUSION: Ever since I first found out that Barbara had breast cancer, the thought of her dying plagued me almost daily. I never told her how I felt about this because I tried to be her coach and source of strength. There were many nights, especially when she was in the hospital with the infections, that I cried myself to sleep. I just kept thinking that it was so unfair for her to have cancer and suffer all the humiliation and sickness that came with the chemotherapy treatments. I never really got over the fear of losing her. I was so afraid of what would happen to me. How could I go on with my life without her? How would I cope with never seeing her or talking with her again? I thought a lot about death during this period. I firmly believed in the afterlife and eternal salvation. I knew that Barbara was a good Christian and that her place in heaven would be a certainty. But I wanted her here on earth with me for the rest of my life. I wanted to see her grow old and comfort me. I couldn't stand the thought of her dying before me. After all, I was the one who served in the Army, a very dangerous profession that, at any minute, could have thrust me in harm's way to face the strong possibility of death.

I woke up every day with gut-wrenching anxiety attacks. I didn't sleep well and would often awake in the middle of the night in fear and confusion. I felt so helpless and so sorry for my poor wife who faced each new problem with a smile and a positive attitude. I knew all along that she was afraid, but she did a good job of hiding it. I guess that this attitude helped give me some strength in my lonely world full of confusion and pain.

SOME THINGS I DID AND SOME THINGS I COULD HAVE DONE: Barbara received her treatment for breast cancer at the University of Kansas Cancer Center, a research and teaching institution. This had a lot of benefits for us in that they seemed to have the latest information available. Early on the staff provided documents, phone numbers, and addresses where additional information could be obtained. If in doubt about where to go to get information, the

National Cancer Institute located in Bethesda, Maryland—1-800-4-CANCER, www.cancer.gov—is always a good source. They publish hundreds of pamphlets on every type of cancer. In addition to publishing highly educational information about the many forms of the disease, they also publish materials that help family members deal with cancer. The materials are all published in both English and Spanish.

I also found an organization called Y-ME National Breast Cancer Organization, a national organization for breast cancer information and support located in Homewood, Illinois, 1-800-221-2141, www.y-me.org. This organization publishes a bimonthly newsletter with some very useful information.

In all of my research and desire to become knowledgeable about the treatment of breast cancer, I never forgot to look out for myself. I was in excellent physical condition; however, anxiety and lack of sleep eventually took their toll. In hindsight, I should have befriended someone to look after my health, too. They could have served as a sounding board and provided feedback about my physical and emotional condition. Also, I should have sought out a cancer support group, even if Barbara did not want to attend. By going to regular meetings I might have found a place to release some of my emotions in addition to finding another venue from which to gather facts.

QUEST FOR KNOWLEDGE: One of the hardest things that I found out early on was learning about breast cancer and then trying to educate my family and friends. To educate myself I spent some time in the public library doing some reading and research. I studied all I could get my hands on that explained the effects of cancer. I studied anatomy books and became very knowledgeable about the function of most of the major organs of the body. I also became familiar with a lot of the medical jargon and definitions of drugs, what they were supposed to do if taken properly, and all of the side effects that could occur. I called the toll-free numbers to the American Institute for Cancer Research, 1-800-843-8114, the National Cancer Institute, 1-800-422-6237 and any local organizations I could find for information. I read and studied all the pamphlets from the Cancer Center in Kansas City and from the Army hospital in Fort Leavenworth. In short, I tried to become as knowledgeable as I could on the thing that was trying to take away my wife. I suppose it was not too different from the training that I received in the military. If you are going to destroy an enemy, then the more you know about him the better your chances become for success.

In summary, here is what I learned from all my studies: Every human being has DNA that makes up his or her genetic code. The most important task for our DNA is to control cell division. Within our DNA there are oncogenes and tumor-suppresser genes, which normally operate together to control cell growth. However if there are defects in these genes caused either by radiation, viruses, environmental poisons, or bad genes inherited from parents, then these cells can grow into tumors. Theses tumors can split again and again, creating even more malignant tumors. These malignant cells develop their own capillaries that provide them with nutrients. The malignant tumors ward off the body's natural defense system (white blood cells). Once secured, the cancer cells use the body's circulatory and lymphatic systems to travel to other parts of the body and create new malignant tumors. This is known as metastasizing. At the time that I studied this deadly disease, there were only three ways to fight against cancer: surgery, radiation, and chemotherapy. I also leaned that the breast contains a lot of fatty tissue and that cancer cells like to seek out fatty cells. Much to my disappointment, I also found out that inflammatory carcinoma of the breast was the most lethal of all the varieties of breast cancer.

SHOCK AND FOCUS: During the initial stages of Barbara's treatment in late 1992, I was in shock. It all seemed so unreal, like a bad nightmare. But it was no dream. It was real and events were moving along quickly. It was during this period that I also felt a change come over me. I had always been sort of a materialistic individual. But my attitude toward those things began to change. I had to keep focus and concentrate on managing the treatment of my wife. The most important thing in the world was Barbara, her well being and receiving the best possible treatment to enhance the probability of a successful recovery. Material objects, money, and work all took a backseat. Nothing mattered except Barbara and our joint fight against cancer. My life had been altered so drastically, that I often found that I did things out of the ordinary that I never would have done in the past.

GETTING ORGANIZED: After our first visit to the Cancer Center, I quickly realized that I needed a planning calendar where I could keep track of Barbara's treatment schedule and the type and amount of drugs that she had to take. I supplemented this with the maintenance of a daily and, in some cases hourly, journal. I recorded every little detail to include attitudes, emotions, type, and amount of drugs, start and stop time of Barbara's period, eating habits, problems of all sorts like lack of bowel movement or aches and pains. I wrote down everything that I observed, and then put it into my computer for a permanent record. This detailing of events paid off big in a couple of tight situations. I always accompanied Barbara to the hospital for her doctor appointments and chemotherapy treatments. When she was admitted to the ER with the infection problems I was able to describe in full detail the type and amount of drugs that she was currently receiving. This helped the doctors and it kept me informed as to exactly what was going on, making me feel like I still had some sort of control. I also added a closing paragraph each day to my journal that described how I felt. I simply called it "emotions." In this paragraph I jotted down how things had gone for me throughout the day. I found this very useful because it helped me vent some of the frustration that I kept built up inside.

MY THERAPY: In the initial months of December 1992 and January 1993, I really didn't do much except keep the house cleaned, cook on occasion, go to work and look after Barbara's needs. She told me at one point that I was hovering too close and that I needed to back off and give her some space. She spent the majority of both day and night in bed. So I felt an obligation to be ready at her calling to get Kleenex or water or juice or whatever she needed. In essence, I had turned into her day-and-night nurse, cook, and counselor. But she was right; she was sick but not helpless. So I took her advice and started to work in my workshop building her a new cherry wood kitchen table. Woodworking was a new hobby and I was still in the learning stages. I found, however, that concentrating on the task of building something took my mind off things even though it was only for a short period.

BITTERNESS AND PAIN: No matter how hard I tried, I couldn't get rid of the thought that this horrible disease just might claim her life. Here we were, forty-four years of age, close to retirement from the Army, and our sons were both grown and just about out of college. This was the prime of our lives when we should be setting goals and objectives for the retirement years. We should have been dreaming about vacations without kids, and discussing how we would treat our yet unborn grandchildren. Instead, we went from doctor to doctor, hospital to hospital and I watched them pump lots of drugs into my sweetheart's body trying to destroy a killer disease. I was becoming a bitter person. I felt that life was unfair. I hated cancer and I hated the chemotherapy that was destroying Barbara's body. Why couldn't we find the cause of breast cancer? Then she wouldn't have to suffer.

FACING REALITY: On the way to the hospital one morning, I had a huge lump in my throat and tears in my eyes. I was tired and stressed. I came to the realization that no matter how much I prayed and monitored Barbara's treatment, if she was going to die from breast cancer there was nothing that I could do to stop it. That really didn't take away the anxiety of knowing that I might lose my best friend, but it did help me come to grips with human vulnerability and the lack of "magic modern medicine."

DEALING WITH MY SPOUSE: It would be too simple to say that Barbara and I had a perfect marriage, but it is probably the closest to the truth as I can get. We literally never fought in twenty-five years of marriage. We had disagreements, but we worked them out quickly. We complemented each other tremendously. I always tried to treat her like the beauty queen that she was. Even after twenty-five years of marriage, I still opened the door for her, held her coat while she put it on and generally tried to be a proper gentleman. Our sex life had grown and enriched over the years. Neither of us ever cheated on the other and we were able to maintain a bond of love and trust that got us through some pretty hard times in our life together. We did change our sexual frequencies during the treatment for cancer. I won't go into any details except that it was something that we discussed early, right after the effects of the first chemotherapy treatment were known. Barbara was tired most of the time. She exhibited little energy and had no desire for sexual activities. For me this was OK. I told her that her health was more important.

DEALING WITH FAMILY: Telling my sons that their mother had a serious form of cancer was no easy task. Tom, the older, was sympathetic and understanding and basically felt that his mother was a strong woman and that she had the willpower and strength to win her battle with breast cancer. Jason, our younger, was very close to his mother. Like his brother, he was sympathetic and understanding. Like me he hated the idea that his mother was sick. He just wanted the doctors to fix her up so she could return to being good old Mom.

I was never successful in convincing the rest of my family that breast cancer was a serious and deadly disease. My parents and brothers and sisters were all supportive, but I am not sure that they really understood how quickly breast cancer could kill a woman. I know that they had no idea how horribly sick Barbara became after the chemotherapy treatments. They only saw Barbara when she was feeling halfway decent or in between chemotherapy treatments. I think to them chemotherapy was more like the cure-all for the cancer, like taking an aspirin to get rid of a headache. But I knew that the harsh effects of the chemotherapy were literally sapping the life out of my wife.

Barbara's parents and family lived on the East Coast in Cape Cod. She had one sister who lived in Phoenix, Arizona. They were all loving and caring with lots of phone calls and flowers and cards in support, but they never saw her during the treatment. So I am not so sure that they really knew how sick Barbara was during this time.

One person who did understand our predicament was my best friend, Jack O'Connor, who also lived in Phoenix. Jack was a retired lieutenant colonel from the Army. We had known each other since we were sixteen and in high school. During his Army stint, Jack earned a doctorate degree in exercise physiology, and his wife, Ellen, was an Intensive Care Unit nurse. I am sure that over the years that she had seen her fair share of cancer patients in the ICU. Jack called me often to offer words of encouragement. Jack and Ellen were both concerned. Jack offered to help check out the Cancer Center in Kansas City. He said that he had some friends in the medical profession and he would call them to get their opinion. I guess that he just wanted to help, so I agreed. A few days later he called me back and reported that the hospital and their staff in Kansas City had a very good reputation.

DEALING WITH FRIENDS AND COWORKERS: My friends at work were sympathetic, but there really wasn't anything that they could do to help out no matter how many times they offered. They did remain supportive and always visited Barbara in the hospital and sent flowers every time she was admitted.

My boss at the time was understanding and he told me that nothing was more important than the health of my wife and that I should take whatever time I needed to be with her when she required it.

On many days I would sit around at work and discuss Barbara's progress with my coworkers. They were all concerned not only for Barbara, but for my welfare as well. There wasn't a day that went by that someone didn't ask me how things were going. I told them the facts as I knew them and always tried to project a positive attitude no matter how bad I felt. I was never afraid to show my emotions to anyone, but I had such faith and hope that somehow we were going to beat cancer.

DEALING WITH GOD: I had always tried to live a good Christian life. Both Barbara and I were raised Roman Catholic and we had a good moral upbringing. We raised our sons in the Catholic faith and most of my family and truly great friends were practicing Christians. So I didn't have a problem dealing with God because I had always dealt with him in my own way. I prayed a lot and always remembered the meaning of the words "Thy will be done" in the Lord's Prayer. Every time I said that prayer I knew that if I really meant it, then I must be willing to accept whatever God did. That is not to say that I put the whole thing in his hands. Nor did I ever feel that God zapped Barbara with cancer for some evil that she had done, or that he was testing our strength. I simply came to realize that Barbara had a horrible affliction and if the doctors and all of the drugs couldn't save her life, then it was in God's hands. I did and still believe in miracles and that is where "Thy will be done" comes in so vividly. It was not up to the doctors, me, family, friends, or even Barbara's positive attitude and strong will to survive. If God wanted to interfere and cure her, then it was his will and not any-one else's.

DEALING WITH MYSELF: Throughout my entire life I had always been a problem solver. I worked hard to get resolution to everything. I was not always successful in getting the resolution that I wanted, and I made mistakes of judgment on occasion. I enjoyed a hard challenge and took great pleasure when I completed a task. But the challenge of helping your wife beat cancer was something that I never thought I would have to face. It just always seemed that since we were such a happily married couple that communicated well, that we would go on to the golden years together. I had a difficult time knowing that I couldn't do a thing to cure Barbara from cancer. All I could do was fight with her and provide as much comfort and support as I could. I did a lot of soul searching and philosophical pondering about the meaning of life in general. I found that I had a hard time focusing on anything but the battle with cancer. It was consuming. It occupied my every thought. But during this time I also found that I had strengths that I didn't know. When you are at your lowest ebb in your life, somehow you find the strength to carry on with your life. I found that I was much more pleasant with people than I ever had been before. At the same time, I found myself wishing that someone else had my problems. I would see couples in perfect health and ask, "Why not them?" Not that I really wanted them to have cancer, but I just wanted it taken away from us. I guess that I was just really angry and bitter that others had the perfect life that I once had.

During this time of anger, bitterness, sorrow, depression, and hatred of what we had been dealt, I never gave up hope. Only one look at my beautiful wife was all that I needed to keep me going strong and hoping for the best. Her spirit and character gave me such strength and courage. She faced the cancer with complete confidence that one day it would all be over and we could get back to the happy routine that we both cherished so much. Granted it would be a different life, because we would always live with the fear that the cancer would come back. But we vowed to each other that we would take it one step at a time. And the saddest part of it all was that we had very few choices except to do exactly what we were doing at the time. There is no magic cure when dealing with cancer.

5

SURGERY, RECOVERY, AND ADJUNCT CHEMOTHERAPY

During the first week of February 1993, Barbara still didn't have a lot of energy. She did force herself to get out of bed and try to complete some small household chores. In the meantime, I kept up with most of the house chores. On occasion a friend would bring by a casserole dish, which we both appreciated very much. As the month went along and she got farther from the time of the last Cytoxan pill, Barbara slowly started to recover. She took a few rides with my parents looking at new housing construction and the new Wal-Mart store in Leavenworth.

On the February 3, Barbara asked me to call Dr. Combs and ask him to put in a Hickman catheter. She had talked to several other cancer patients, and they all told her that the catheter was the best way to go. Her arms were a mess from all of the needle sticks and her veins were shrinking as a result of the chemotherapy. I called the doctor, and he told me that he would not recommend it unless Barbara's oncologist, Dr. Ramos, wanted it. Apparently he had some bad experience in the past with the Hickman and just didn't want to risk anything that would cause more infection. Barbara was upset over his decision.

On February 8, I was unable to take Barbara to KU Cancer Center for the beginning of her fourth cycle of chemotherapy, so my parents gladly escorted her. During the exam with Dr. Ramos, he remarked how good the site around the tumor looked. He told Barbara that he felt that the chemotherapy was really attacking the tumor and that she was ready for the surgery. So Barbara did not receive a treatment. She was glad that she didn't have to have another treatment that day. Dr. Ramos told Barbara to make an appointment to see him two weeks after she had the surgery.

When I got home that evening and she told me the news, we sat down and discussed the upcoming operation. Neither of us felt badly about her losing a breast. We both knew that the breast contained the source of all her problems.

She asked me how I felt. My response came in the form of a demonstration. I told her to suppose I had an accident at work that required the removal of one of my arms. I then put my left arm behind my back and asked her if she would love me any less if I only had one arm. Of course her response was no. So I told her that was the way I felt about her losing a breast. The next day she called Dr. Combs and set the appointment for the operation for February 17, 1993.

Dr. Combs was good in describing to me the exact procedure. Barbara was to undergo a modified radical mastectomy. He said that he would remove the breast and the lymph nodes under her right arm, leaving the pectoral muscle in place and only removing the protective cover over the top of the muscle.

The morning of the operation arrived and we got up at 5:30 AM to get ready to go to the hospital. After the usual check-in procedure, Barbara was ready to go to the operating room. At 7:18 AM Barbara walked down the same hallway that she walked down for the biopsy operation. I went to the same set of fixed chairs along the wall of the third floor of Munson Army Health Center. My mother arrived around 8:00 AM to keep me company during the operation. We sat, drank some coffee, talked a little, and waited for the surgeon to come out and tell us how the operation went. Dr. Combs came out of the operating room around 11:30 AM. He said that he felt very good about the operation and that Barbara was doing well in the recovery room. About forty-five minutes later, they wheeled her out of the recovery room toward her room in the hospital. Barbara looked tired and told me that she wanted something to drink. The nurses said that it was not a good idea because of the effects of the anesthesia. So I got her some ice to suck on until she was capable of drinking fluids. The nurses brought her some Percocet for pain relief. I had to admit that she looked a lot better than I thought she would, but Barbara was a beautiful woman, and she looked good no matter what the circumstances.

Barbara's recovery in the hospital only lasted seven days. She had a remarkable knack for healing quickly. During this time she received a lot of cards, phone calls, and flowers. She was truly loved by friends and family. I went back to my routine of stopping by in the morning before work and spending lunch with her in the afternoon. The visits from friends and family really seemed to help her spirits. She was sore from the operation but loved people stopping by for a short visit. On her last day in the hospital, Dr. Combs took out the drainage tubes from the area around the incision. In Barbara's words, "It hurt like hell." I asked the doctor why he used staples to close the incision. He told me that they were quicker and tighter, leaving less of a scar. After our conversation, he released her from the hospital and told her to come back in two more weeks to get the staples removed. When we got home we both examined the area of the surgery and determined that it wasn't too bad and that the doctor had done a very good job. We went back to the hospital on February 26, and Dr. Combs removed the staples. Now it was time to call the oncologist and set up an appointment to resume the dreaded adjunct chemotherapy. Barbara got an appointment for March 10, so she'd have a little more time to recover from the operation and get her strength back before getting more chemotherapy.

The days and weeks after the operation were very good times for both of us, but particularly for Barbara. She absolutely hated the idea of getting more chemotherapy but she knew that it had to be done. On the day of the oncology appointment, Barbara received a call from Dr. Combs. He told her that during the operation he had removed eight lymph nodes and the results of the pathology report only showed traces of cancer cells in one of the nodes. We were elated with the news. In our previous conversations with the oncology nurses and from my research, we knew that if she had a lot of lymph nodes infected with cancer that it meant that there was a pretty good probability that the cancer had spread to other parts of the body. With only one of the eight nodes infected, we felt that there was a much better chance that the cancer had been contained, and removed with the operation. We had great hope for a full recovery.

6

MORE CHEMOTHERAPY

On March 10 we went back to the Cancer Center to begin the adjunct chemotherapy. Dr. Ramos commented on how good Barbara looked after the surgery. It had been forty-six days since she took her last dose of chemotherapy. After the exam, Dr. Ramos said that he wanted Barbara to go through six more cycles of chemotherapy. I told him that she already had completed three and asked why she needed six more when he initially said that the total would be six cycles. He said the three cycles before the operation did not count toward adjunct therapy and that she needed at least six more cycles to ensure that any remaining microscopic cancer cells would be destroyed. I looked at Barbara and saw the devastating disappointment in her eyes. We thought that we would be through with all of this by June, and now they were telling us that it would be sometime at the end of the summer if all went well. Barbara and I discussed the dosage with Dr. Ramos and convinced him to reduce everything by 25 percent. He did some quick calculations and rewrote the prescription for all of the chemotherapy drugs. The nurses then administered the first adjunct chemotherapy treatment.

The majority of March was a much better time for Barbara. The reduction in the chemotherapy, particularly the Cytoxan, seemed to give her just a little more energy. Her hair had started to grow back in the forty-six days of no chemotherapy and we noticed that it was about the same color as before. That was good news; some cancer patients never grow their hair back. At this point every little positive sign was welcomed.

On March 26 Barbara and my mother drove to Kansas City to get fitted for a mastectomy prosthesis. She was gone most of the day and, by the time she got home, I was home from work sitting on our deck drinking a beer. Barbara came outside after greeting our two Schnauzers and twirled around like a ballerina. She was showing off her new "breast." I told her that it looked really good and she responded that it made her feel whole again. She took me in the house and took off the prosthesis to show me how it worked. This model was the kind that had

Velcro strips on the back. She had to glue the receptive side of the Velcro in a horseshoe shape on her chest and simply attach the breast. This meant that she could wear her own bras. It was so nice to see her smiling and showing some pride in her appearance. She really was looking pretty good despite the weight that she had started to put on as a result of fluid retention caused by the chemotherapy.

Barbara continued to stay in close contact with her family. Her sister, Sue, was getting married in Phoenix in September and wanted Barbara to be the matron of honor. We agreed that depending on her physical state at that point, it would be a nice break to go away for a short vacation. Barbara's parents also stayed in constant touch. At this point she felt so good that the tumor had been removed and that she only had three more cycles of chemotherapy to go through. Her spirits were high and hopes for recovery looked promising.

We both tried not to reflect on the previous months and how lousy she felt. We decided that the events of the past were just that—past. It was something that we went through together and they were over. We were always looking forward to healing and a better life. We tried to go on with events in our lives in as normal a way as possible. On one occasion Barbara accompanied me to the Ford dealer to pick up her 1991 Probe that was in the shop for some small repairs. I was around back settling some insurance papers when one of the salesmen stuck his head in the door and said that my wife wanted to see me. I told him to tell her to come in, that I was just about finished. He insisted that I come outside to see her. When I opened the door, there sat Barbara in the driver's seat of a brand new 1993 Rio Red Ford Probe GT. She said, "Don't I look good in this? Let's take it for a drive!" We left the dealership as proud owners of a new car.

On April 5, 1993, we arrived at the Cancer Center for the second treatment of adjunct chemotherapy. Once again we were told that Barbara's white blood cell count was too low to administer the drugs. We made another appointment for the following week and told the nurses to call before we drove all the way to Kansas City if there were any problems. When we returned the next week, three different oncology nurses failed to find a vein in Barbara's arm. The problem was exacerbated because they could now only use her left arm for needle sticks. With the removal of the lymph nodes under her right arm, she didn't have much of a drainage system on that side. The right arm could only be used if it were an emergency. Nurse Barbara called Dr. Ramos and recommended that he call Dr. Combs to discuss allowing Barbara to have a Hickman catheter emplaced. Everyone agreed and we decided to have it done at the University of Kansas Medical

Center, which was in the same building as the Cancer Center. The surgery was scheduled for April 12.

So on a nice spring morning in April 1993, we found ourselves in the hospital for the placement of the catheter. We both thought that this would be a relatively simple procedure with no risks and a lot of benefits, namely no more needles in the arms. But after talking to the surgeon and listening to the dangers of the operation and of the potential for infection, I had a much different picture in my mind. After several attempts to insert the needle by the nurses failed, an anesthesiologist was able to get the butterfly IV in Barbara's arm so that they could administer the anesthesia. The doctor was successful because he could use prescription drug lidocaine to deaden the area in the arm where he eventually managed to stick the butterfly IV.

Barbara was in the operating room for about forty-five minutes and another hour was spent in the recovery room. The doctor came out and told me that everything went well and gave me a brief explanation about the function of the Hickman. Simply stated, it was nothing more than a thin surgical line placed into the patient's subclavian vein. This is the vein that runs under the breastbone and close to the heart. The Hickman had an exit site just to the right of the patient's breast with a Y junction where two lines with caps were attached. It was at these two ports that the nurses could administer injections and draw blood.

Barbara got dressed and we walked over to the Cancer Center to begin the second adjunct chemotherapy treatment. We had to sit in the treatment center for four hours instead of the usual hour. The nurses explained that they had to use heparin (an anticoagulant) longer the first time using the Hickman to ensure that the newly implanted lines were clear. Barbara and I watched a video about the care and treatment of the catheter. After her chemotherapy treatment we left the center with a bag full of supplies, all for the catheter.

The next day a home care nurse stopped by to see Barbara and changed the dressing around the catheter. She later called me to see if I could meet her around noon the next day at our house so she could watch me do all of the things that I supposedly learned from the video. In the meantime, Barbara went to the Army hospital to the physical therapy ward. The therapists told her that her right arm and the area around the breast removal looked real good, and that it was obvious that Barbara had routinely completed her exercises as instructed.

The next day at noon I met the home care nurse and proceeded to change the dressing and flush out the two ports on the Hickman. It took me about ten minutes and beside some minor corrections, the nurse said that I did a fine job. I went back to work and Barbara went shopping with my mother and sister.

The month of May was pretty much the same as April. Barbara completed another adjunct chemotherapy treatment and generally felt pretty good. On June 4 we went to our older son's college graduation. It was really a very nice time. Barbara by now had gained about thirty pounds with the chemotherapy, but she still had the beauty and charm that could overwhelm anyone. It was a hot day and I know that she was very hot with her wig. I could see the sweat pouring down the sides of her face. I watched her closely and made sure that she had plenty of fluids to drink. After the long, three-hour graduation ceremony in the hot sun, we went to one of the local taverns for some food and beer. Around 7:00 PM I could see that Barbara was tired, so we excused ourselves and left for home. All in all it was a good day for the both of us. Young Tom was the first of the Brown grandchildren to graduate from college. Barbara was beaming with pride all day long.

Barbara completed her fourth adjunct chemotherapy on June 21, her fifth on July 20, and the final cycle on August 18. This now totaled eight months of chemotherapy. By now she had put on about forty pounds of extra weight and really looked bloated. But we were elated that it was finally over. The last checkup with the doctor in August went well and he told her to come back in September after we returned from her sister's wedding. He also recommended a schedule of close follow-ups to include a complete physical exam every six months with a mammogram. After a year of this, the mammogram could then be conducted yearly. He made no bones at all about the seriousness of inflammatory breast cancer. When we asked where it was likely to recur, he said that it could come back anywhere in her body but there was a good probability it would seek out the brain as a likely depository. Barbara knew the risks and lived in constant fear that it would come back, but decided that all was clear for now and that she would get on with her life.

7

THE WEDDING AND ANOTHER BOUT WITH INFECTION

We left for sister Sue's wedding on September 2, 1993. It was a great flight out to Phoenix, and it was real nice to see her sister again. We met Frank DeGeorge, Sue's fiancé, and they took us to our hotel room. We stayed at The Pointe in Squaw Valley, a very ritzy place. The weather was beautiful and warm. For the first couple of days, we had leisurely breakfasts and spent time sitting around the pool enjoying the company of her sister and the sunshine.

The day before the wedding, I had a golf outing scheduled with my best friend, Jack O'Connor. Barbara's dad, Robert, who was seventy-nine at the time, also went along with us to play. We drove for about an hour to get to the Tournament Players Course in Scottsdale, Arizona, which is the first stop on the PGA tour. It was a great day and very hot, about 110 degrees. We had two carts and plenty of ice and water. On the back nine Robert started feeling a little down from the heat. Jack and I told him to take a cart and go to the clubhouse, but he said that he was fine, that he would just ride along and watch us finish out the round.

On the way home from the golf course, Robert started really feeling ill. He was sitting in the backseat of the car and I told him to lie down. He was moaning by now and his skin was pale and cool to the touch. We were about ten minutes away from the hotel. Occasionally he would prop himself back up and appear to be OK. When we arrived at the hotel he said that he felt much better. So we all got out of the car and started to walk toward the elevator of the hotel. Just as we got to the foyer, he said that he needed to sit down for a minute. As soon as he sat down he collapsed. Jack immediately went into first aid, loosening his collar and getting a towel wet from a nearby fountain. Since we were in the rear parking lot of the hotel, I knew that I could get to the phone in my room quicker than running around the building to the lobby. I ran up to my room and called the hotel lobby for an ambulance. To my surprise, John and Pam, Barbara's youngest brother and sister-in-law, were up in the room with Aileen, Barbara's mother. They had just flown in from Cape Cod to surprise Sue for the wedding. I told them about Bob and John, Aileen, Pam, and Barbara all rushed down to see what they could do. The hotel medics had arrived by the time I got back. Soon an ambulance team was on the scene, and Barbara's father was rushed off to the hospital.

We all followed the ambulance to the hospital. The doctors diagnosed a slight case of dehydration and heat exhaustion. After several hours of IV drips, he was released, and we all returned to the hotel. It was a scary event, and we all felt much more comfortable once we knew that the old man was going to be all right.

By the next evening Robert was feeling much better. Barbara's aunt and uncle arrived from Flagstaff, Arizona, in the afternoon and we had a few drinks and a lot of laughs before we left for the church. The wedding came and went in the usual style. Both Barbara and Sue looked beautiful up on the altar as the minister went through the ceremony. I knew that Barbara was tired but she stood through the entire event and never faltered once. We stayed at the reception for quite a while and then left for the hotel. Jack O'Connor and I had planned another golf match the next day.

On Sunday morning Barbara and I got up early and went down to the hotel restaurant for breakfast. The waiter brought us some ice water, took our order and left. Barbara sipped the water and waited for her order to come. We talked about the wedding and how beautiful the weather and the hotel were. Soon the breakfast arrived and we started to eat. I noticed that Barbara was shivering. I asked her what was wrong and she just responded that she was cold. She thought that the ice water had given her a chill. The shaking got worse and I told her to go stand outside in the sun to try to warm up. After several minutes of her not returning I left some money for the bill and went out to find her. She didn't look good at all and had uncontrollable shaking. I took her back up to the hotel room and got the blanket off the bed and wrapped her up. I felt her forehead to see if I could detect any fever. I told her that she felt a little warm to me and that I was going out to find a thermometer to take her temperature. I also told her that I was going to call Jack and cancel the golf match. In her typical unselfish fashion, she insisted that she would be all right and that I should go on to play golf with Jack. But I knew better. I knew that something was not right and I kept thinking back to the two previous stays in the hospital that were all the result of a low white blood cell count and an infection somewhere.

I got in the rental car and drove to Walgreen's and purchased a thermometer. When I got back to the hotel Barbara was no better. I took her temperature and found it to be 102.2 degrees. I told her that we needed to go to the local hospital to get checked out. Barbara just smiled and told me that she would be all right. She insisted that I should go on with Jack and play golf. I waited another hour and saw that she was not getting any better. By the time I convinced Barbara that she needed to go to the hospital, she was too weak to stand. I went to the phone, called the lobby, and told them that my wife was ill and that she needed an ambulance. When the ambulance crew arrived, I pulled out my charts and told them all of her past medical history, including the last drugs taken during chemotherapy. The paramedics went through the usual checks and then loaded her in the ambulance for the trip to the hospital. I followed in the rental car and went into the admissions office to file the appropriate forms for our insurance company. In a short time, I demanded to be taken to the ER room so that I could be with my wife. When I finally was escorted to Barbara's bedside I asked her how she felt. She responded with her usual smile, but her face showed a great deal of disappointment. She was blaming herself for ruining our short vacation in Arizona.

The attending physician asked me about her medical history. He was concerned about the high temperature. He directed the nursing staff to try to break the fever with Tylenol. So, here we were once again back in the familiar surroundings of the hospital room with another problem yet to be defined. I told the doctor that I was in the Army, and, if there was any military facility nearby, then we needed to evacuate her to the military hospital. He made a call to the nearest Air Force Base some thirty miles away. After several minutes of conversation, he told me that the duty doctor authorized him to admit Barbara into the Phoenix hospital.

After several vials of blood were drawn for culture tests, Barbara was finally moved out of the ER ward to a hospital room. I stayed with her waiting for some kind of word from the doctor's diagnosis. The attending physician ordered a general antibiotic to fight off infection until he could get the results of the culture tests that would supposedly isolate the source of the infection. I called back to the hotel to let everyone know Barbara's status as soon as she was admitted.

When I was sure that she was resting comfortably, I drove back to the hotel to make some arrangements. I called my secretary back at Fort Leavenworth and told her to extend my leave time. I contacted the hotel reservations desk and asked them to extend our reservations by one week, and I left the return flight open with the airlines. Everyone was very cooperative. I had some supper, talked to Barbara's parents for a while and then went back to the hospital.

The next day, the attending physician stopped by to examine Barbara again. Barbara's condition remained about the same. She was still running a fever, and the doctor felt about 90 percent sure that the Hickman catheter was the source of the infection, although her temperature was being controlled with the Tylenol. He told us it needed to come out. We asked him why he came to that conclusion. He said that the symptoms that Barbara was demonstrating were similar to situations that he had seen in other patients. Barbara and I both agreed that if he was so sure, then the catheter should be removed. The doctor made arrangements with a surgeon to come to the room to remove the Hickman.

The surgeon didn't arrive until around 4:30 PM. He brought in a couple of nurses to assist in the procedure. They pulled Barbara's gown away from her chest and she lay there fully exposed with her one remaining breast. I saw that the door to the room was still open and that any passersby could easily see what was going on. So I walked over and closed the door and made a comment to all present that they should be a little more considerate of privacy. I guess that doctors and nurses in hospitals see so much that they often forget to be considerate of the patient's privacy.

The surgeon gave Barbara several shots of lidocaine to deaden the area around the Hickman. I know that it hurt like hell and burned. He then made a small incision above the exit site of the catheter ports and began to look inside for the line. When he found the line, he began looking for a small felt cuff that went around the line to prevent it from slipping and coming out if pulled too hard. He had a hard time getting the line removed because skin tissue was growing around it. He cut the line in half, removed the felt cuff, and pulled the top part out from the new incision, and the remainder of the line was pulled from the exit site. He cleaned the area, put in several stitches, and the nurses applied a dressing. The whole procedure took about fifteen minutes.

A day later we got the word back from the attending physician that the Hickman was indeed infected and was the cause of what turned out to be a staph infection. Barbara didn't remember, but only a few months before I had lost a good friend at age fifty-two from a staph infection. Staphylococcus is a nasty killer bacteria that can spread quickly in the human body if it is unchecked by antibiotics. With a little research I found out that staph infections can invade and attack any part of your body, from your skin, eyes, and nails to the inner lining of your heart. The symptoms vary, depending on where the infection develops. Staph infections usually enter the body through an open cut or wound. The infection can spread to adjacent tissue or, through the bloodstream, to internal organs such as the heart or kidneys, where it can become life threatening. People with a chronic illness such as diabetes, cancer, or chronic liver or kidney disease, or those who inject illegal drugs, are particularly susceptible to severe staph infections. A person who suspects a staph infection should look for the following signs:

- Pain and swelling around a cut or scraped area of skin.

- Boils or small, white-headed pimples around hair follicles.

- In infants and young children, blistering and peeling skin.

- Swollen lymph nodes in the neck, armpits, or groin.

When I arrived at the hospital the next day and greeted my wife, she started crying. I asked her what was wrong and she held up her left hand. I looked at her wedding rings and noticed that the diamond stone was missing. She was really upset and said that she didn't know where it had fallen out and that she had just noticed it. We both thought that she might have snagged it on the blankets during her sleep. So we took the bed apart and looked everywhere to no avail. So much had happened in the past twenty-four hours, to lose her diamond, too, was more than her worn-out psyche could handle. No wonder she had been crying. I felt badly for her and comforted her by telling her that we would replace the stone. This seemed to help a little, but I know that she felt a very special attachment for something that she had worn for over twenty-four years.

Barbara remained in the hospital for several more days, receiving large doses of antibiotics to clear up the infection. Finally the fever went away, and she began to feel much better. She was now ready to get out of the hospital. The doctor did not want to release her but she demanded to go. He gave in and prescribed some oral antibiotics to be taken and ordered her to see Dr. Combs immediately upon her return to Leavenworth. We went back to the hotel, checked out, drove to the airport, turned in the rental car, and boarded our flight for the return trip. On our way back to Leavenworth, I told Barbara how scared I was with her bout with the staph infection in Phoenix. I confessed to her that I really didn't think she was going to make it through the hospital stay. She did not have any idea how sick she really was and how fast that type of infection can consume a human body. The look on her face was one of love and concern. She hugged me, gave me a soft kiss, and thanked me for my support. I felt gratified, but still helpless to cure her from that terrible disease. I knew that our life together would never be a normal one again. The thought of another tumor appearing somewhere remained in my mind. But I remembered the vows that I took, in particular the part about "in sickness and in health." I renewed that vow again in my mind, as I knew we had many more challenges ahead.

8

A NEW BEGINNING

Back in our home, we had a fresh beginning. Barbara had gotten rid of the tumor, lost a breast, the Hickman was removed, and she was finished with chemotherapy. We resumed our daily routines and she got farther away from the effects of the chemotherapy, I could see her slowly regaining her strength. Her spirits were lifted, and we both watched with great anticipation as her hair started to grow back. At first it seemed to grow very quickly, but it soon slowed. We had a nightly ritual where I would massage her scalp. She thought that it would help her hair to return more rapidly. I didn't mind giving her massages, considering all the crap that she had put up with over the past ten months. In fact the ritual extended from the rubbing of the head to a total body massage finishing with her feet.

Barbara began to regain her strength, and she appeared to have an interest in an active sex life again. Our lovemaking at first was slow and infrequent. But after awhile she gained more strength and desire and things were getting back to what we both considered somewhat normal. That is to say a normal sex life for a couple that had been together for over twenty-four years. I was always gentle with her and kept in mind that she had hidden emotions about the loss of a breast and having very little hair. She told me that she didn't feel very sexy, but I reassured her that my love for her was not based on her physical beauty. It always seemed kind of odd to me that I never really thought of her as any less a woman because she only had one breast, and that she was suffering the common effects of menopause, which included hot flashes and mood swings. I loved her for who she was and, at this time in our lives, I felt extremely grateful that she was still alive for me to love. I know that our bond of love was built over many years of trust and communication. It never stopped. Neither did her physical condition at the time handicap our relationship. We were truly soul mates.

Barbara went back to the KU Cancer Center for another bone and CAT scan in mid-September. The results showed a small polyp on her right lung. When

Dr. Ramos told us of the news, we were shocked and feared the worst. He didn't seem concerned and said that it was a common occurrence for people living in the Missouri Valley region. He explained that it could be caused by a variety of things and said that he would watch it to see if it was growing, but for the moment we should not be overly concerned. When we left the hospital, I could see the fear in Barbara's eyes. She lived with the fear that a tumor would come back somewhere else in her body. Now she had an unusual growth on her lungs. I told her not to read into it too much and just wait to see if anything else developed. My words sounded strong and encouraging, but in my heart and mind I prayed that we didn't have to go through all the treatment business again so soon. I knew that if Barbara could get past the magic five-year mark of no recurrence then her chances for long-term survival were good. Each night I asked God not to let the cancer come back. I also asked him for another thirty-five years of life with my beautiful wife. I don't know why I picked thirty-five, it just seemed that we could live out all of our dreams in that time, and then I would be willing to let her go if it was her time. I just didn't want to let her leave me at age forty-four.

The month of October rolled around, and I had a plot in mind to surprise Barbara on her forty-fifth birthday. I approached her one day and asked her once again how much her wedding rings meant to her. She said, "Well, they mean a lot. You gave them to me." I pressed and said that I understood all of that, but I wanted to know if she would be happy with a replacement. She acknowledged that she could be happy with another ring. That was all that I needed to add fuel to my already burning plot. I went to the Army post shopping exchange and looked at the engagement rings. I was looking for a gold band with a one-carat diamond. This would be a perfect match for the gold wedding band that I had given her for our tenth anniversary. I found the ring that I wanted, bought it, and took it home.

Barbara's birthday was October 21. I took her to the best restaurant in town for a wonderful steak dinner. We went back home and the rest of our family arrived for the traditional cake and ice cream. My sister Lisa had baked a beautiful cake and everyone brought Barbara some nice presents. When she was finished opening the presents, she looked at me and said, "Well what did you get me?" I walked around the table took her left hand and slipped on the engagement ring. Overcome with emotion, we cried, hugged, and kissed. I must admit that not only did she look beautiful; she looked very good with that big rock on her hand. For the rest of the night, she walked around showing off her new diamond. It was a night that I will never forget. For a brief moment I was able to provide her with a tangible expression of my deep love. When I looked at her, however, I realized that she shared my love and that all the diamonds in the world would not mean as much to her as the care and comfort that I provided to her.

Thanksgiving came and Barbara was right back in her usual spirit of entertaining. She prepared a meal for over twenty people. Our family and friends that joined us for dinner were all grateful. It was so pleasing for me to see her in her natural state again. It was a state that always showed genuine love and concern for others. She never thought of herself; she always gave so freely to others.

The Christmas season approached and once again Barbara was filled with joy and enthusiasm. She brought out all of the Christmas decorations and proudly displayed them around our home. We even went out and bought a new artificial tree. It seemed that she wanted to give me and our two sons the best Christmas possible. I feel that she was grateful just to be alive and that she wanted to celebrate Christmas of 1993 with as much love and joy as she could muster.

Our twenty-fifth wedding anniversary came on December 28. We maintained our traditional ritual of going away for the night to a nice hotel. That year we chose the Ritz Carlton in Kansas City, Missouri. We left early, checked into the hotel, had a glass of champagne, and then went walking on the Country Club Plaza. It was a cold day but our warmth came from inside as we walked hand-in-hand through all the stores. We met the rest of my family, minus young Tom who could not make it up from Oklahoma, for a marvelous dinner at a classy restaurant. Tom and Jason had a very special gift for us. They had gone back in some of the old family albums and took certain pictures out and had them enlarged. They put them in a new album and each wrote us a special message. The beginning of the album was a joint message that read, "Today as you are looking back on all the joys you've shared, the many dreams that have come true, the way you both have cared, this brings congratulations and a wish that love and laughter will fill your anniversary and will last forever." At the end of the album Jason wrote, "Mom and Dad, Twenty-five years ago would you believe all that would happen? Including such a great second child? I wouldn't be so great if it weren't for the love and guidance you have given me. Besides congratulations, I would like to say thank you both. I hope that the next sum of years will bring as much happiness as have these past twenty-five. Together we as a family are making our dreams come true every day. I love you both. Happy anniversary, Jason." Our son Tom wrote, "Mom and Dad, I just wanted to say thank you. Thank you for the best twenty-three years of my life. I couldn't ask for more loving, caring, supportive parents. You have definitely brought out the best in me. I am extremely fortunate and very proud to be a part of this family. I think what makes our family so special is the love, trust and support that we all show for each other.

You did good Mom and Dad! Have a great time tonight. I will be thinking about you and again congratulations and thanks. Love #1 Son." I know that the twenty-fifth celebration of a marriage is special, but this night was extra special. We had the love of our sons, family, and friends to share it with us.

After the first of the New Year 1994, Barbara went back to her oncologist for another checkup. The chest X-ray revealed that the polyp on her right lung was gone. We were elated with the news. The doctor's exam also showed her to be in very good health. She was not quite ready to go without the wig, but we knew it wouldn't be long. She also continued her frustrating battle with the extra weight that she had gained. I told her to take it slow, that it had taken a year to put on so it might just take another year to take it back off. She was determined to get back to her normal size, but thanked me just the same for being so considerate of her.

My life at work was pretty normal. By now the almost constant inquiries about my wife's health had ceased. It wasn't that people didn't care anymore; it just seemed that people assumed that Barbara was doing OK. I still received a lot of moral support from friends and family, but the frequencies of their inquiries also slowed down.

One morning in the middle of January 1994, I received a call from my personnel assignment officer in Washington DC. He informed me that in June of that year I would have completed three years at Fort Leavenworth. He added that it would be time for me to move, and he wanted to know what kind of assignment I would like. Knowing the system all too well, I knew that he had some requirements in mind so I asked him what was available. After several more phone calls we narrowed down my choices to two locations. I could either go back to England as the attaché to the U.S. Ambassador or as a faculty member at the U.S. Army War College at Carlisle Barracks, Pennsylvania.

Just like all of my previous assignments, I had lengthy discussions with Barbara about her desires. This move was no different, except we had to worry about her state of health. We both wanted to go back to England. This would be a great job, and it would give us the opportunity to renew friendships that we gained during a previous tour of duty with the Fourth Royal Tank Regiment, British Army of the Rhine from 1983 to 1985. That was a tour that we both enjoyed. However, in our discussions Barbara mentioned that she was concerned about treatment for a cancer recurrence in a foreign country. She also did not want to be too far away from our two sons. With that information in mind, I called my assignment officer and told him I would like to take an assignment to Carlisle Barracks. My assignment officer processed the necessary paperwork for the move, and we started to make preparations.

Housing is always a concern for families in the military because there is always a waiting list for on-post quarters unless you are going somewhere as a direct replacement for someone who is authorized designated housing. Unfortunately, this was not the case on the assignment I received. I called the housing office at Carlisle Barracks and learned that there would be a waiting period of up to a year for a colonel to get quarters. But the lady that I talked with said that it could be possible to receive a smaller set of quarters if we could arrive by mid-April. Since this was several months before my reporting date, I had to get approval from my commanding general to move early. The general gave his approval, and we set things in motion for my replacement at Leavenworth, and travel and household shipping arrangements for the move to Pennsylvania.

Barbara finally felt comfortable enough to go without her wig around the middle of March. Her calendar was constantly full with coffees, lunch, and shopping dates with friends from the fort. She was really back to living the great and wonderful life that she had before the cancer. She had a very busy schedule but seemed to have plenty of energy to carry it out. I was really proud of her enjoying life again after being so sick for the past year. In fact, I even stopped worrying about her health—except in the back of my mind I knew that the evil disease could raise its head at any moment.

My emotions and mental state now were pretty stable. I resumed playing a lot of golf, and working in my shop building furniture. I felt good about the upcoming move and worked hard at my job formulating a plan to easily hand over my position to my replacement.

Our departure from Fort Leavenworth was eminent. We went to several dinner parties in our honor given by friends and family. We tried to spend as much time as we could with our sons. We made frequent trips to Lawrence, Kansas, to visit Jason, and we spent the Easter holiday with Tom in Miami, Oklahoma.

The visits with our sons were very special. Jason took a funny attitude about us moving so far away from Kansas. He liked the convenience of having a home he could go to that was only thirty-nine miles away. We reassured him that we would be available any time he liked, either by phone or a visit if necessary. Tom, who was now in his second year of work after graduating from college, also expressed his concern about us moving. But we were all so happy even though we were moving. The love and trust that had been built up over the years in our family held us together. Little did I know at the time that would be the last time Barbara's sons would see their mother alive.

9

A NEW JOB, A NEW LIFE

April finally arrived, and the arrangements for our departure were just about complete. The only thing left unresolved was where we would live in Carlisle. I kept in constant contact with the housing office at Carlisle Barracks. They told me that a set of quarters would be available if I could arrive there before the eighth of April. On April 6 I left Leavenworth by car. Our plan was for me to drive one car out to Pennsylvania, sign for our quarters, then fly back to Leavenworth and pick up Barbara. In the meantime, Barbara got stuck with the packers and movers in Leavenworth preparing our household goods for shipment. She also inherited the task of cleaning our house and getting it ready to hand over to the renters.

The drive to Carlisle took me two days and I arrived on Thursday evening, April 7. I reported to headquarters the next day and immediately went to the housing office. I was shown a set of quarters on the post. The quarters were adequate. The only problem that remained at this point was that the quarters would not be cleaned and ready for acceptance until April 11. That meant that I had to remain over the weekend before I could sign for the quarters and get the keys. I called the airlines and changed my reservations for an afternoon flight on April 11, back to Kansas. I called Barbara and told her of my plans. She was happy about getting a house so quickly, but frustrated about all the cleaning work that she was doing. Both of my parents were helping Barbara clean our home in Kansas, but it is still a labor-intensive effort. I could tell by her voice and attitude that she was tiring quickly. But in our conversation she did tell me that her last checkup with Dr. Ramos, which included a final bone and CAT scan, went well. She had a clean bill of health for now.

Monday came, and I went and inspected the quarters. After signing the necessary paper work, I left for the airport. I boarded my plane and anxiously waited as we flew across half of the United States. Barbara and my parents picked me up at the airport in Kansas City. We spent our last night together in Kansas and departed early the next morning. Once again, the drive back out to Pennsylvania took us two days. We arrived on April 14. The next day the movers arrived with our household goods and we watched and inventoried as they took all of our belongings off the truck. I remained on leave for the next ten days and helped Barbara unpack all of the boxes. We really worked hard getting everything in place. I watched with great admiration as Barbara arranged our new home. She had a beautiful talent for interior decorating. I was very proud of the work that she did to make our new home a wonderful place to live.

The rest of April, May, and part of June were some of the most pleasant days of our life together. We went out to dinner at many of the local eating establishments, worked on our flower garden and lawn. My new job was exciting and I was just so grateful that Barbara had regained a lot of her self-confidence and pride. She was really losing weight and her head had enough hair by now to get a haircut and styling. I could never understand why her hair meant so much to her. To me she was beautiful, even bald. To her, losing her hair was the most humiliating experience of all that she had been through. For me, when you watch someone go through so much and come so close to death, you overlook the little things like a full head of hair.

Barbara and I took a lot of little short trips. One Saturday I took her to the Gettysburg battlefield for a quick tour. We ended the day eating a good meal at Herr's Tavern, located just outside of Gettysburg, Pennsylvania. Barbara also got right into the community activities at Carlisle. She made new friends and took several day trips to many of the wonderful sites in the surrounding countryside. We both became very good friends with our neighbors. We spent many wonderful nights together in the early summer drinking beer and wine. It seemed to me that we were truly on the road to rebuilding a life that had been so shattered by cancer.

10

RECURRENCE

My parents arrived in Carlisle on June 13 for a two-week visit in our new home. I continued to work for the first week of their visit because Barbara's parents were coming during the second week, and we had many plans. On June 20, Barbara went for her six-month checkup at the Carlisle Barracks Health Clinic. She saw an OB/GYN named Dr. Michael Larson M.D. who gave her a routine exam. Barb asked him to have a blood sample taken because she had been noticing that she was bruising very easily. She also had several boils under her right armpit. One of the boils was large and painful. On Friday evening, June 17, she broke it open and cleaned the site with hydrogen peroxide trying to ward off any form of infection. The results of the blood draw were unusual. Her white blood count was 31,000 (the normal range is between 4,800 and 10,800) and the platelets were 19,000 (the normal range is between 130,000 and 400,000). Because the counts were so erratic, Dr. Larson referred her to a civilian specialist. We made arrangements to see a Dr. Paul Smith M.D. for Tuesday, June 21. The rest of this day and night was not the peace and happiness that we had been experiencing in the past few months. I couldn't stop thinking about all that we had been through together in the last year and a half. Now all of a sudden something was wrong, just after we thought things were really looking good. Barb was deeply depressed. She had such a strong will, but she could just see the whole cancer mess starting all over again. We talked, prayed, and renewed our commitment to fight to the very end.

The next day I got up at 6:30 AM and took our dogs out for a walk. Barb got up about 7:30 and kept herself busy cleaning the house and moving about. She always did this to keep from sitting around and worrying. We left the house about 11:20 AM and drove to see Dr. Smith. The ride to the doctor's office was quiet, as we were both in deep thought about what the results of the visit would be. We saw Dr. Smith together. He had another blood draw and the results were better but still something was wrong. The WBC was 33,000, and the platelets were 60,000; neither of them within the normal range. He conducted a thorough physical exam and seemed intensely concerned about the health of his patient. He looked at the blood smear again and said that he would like to take a couple bone marrow samples before we left. He said that there were early (immature) whites in the blood that indicated there were either too many white cells in the marrow and they were going out into the blood stream too early, or that something was pushing them out before they were mature. Oddly, I think that everyone in the room knew what he referred to when he said "something" was pushing them out. I left the room while he took the sample of bone marrow. He made a slight incision and took a fluid sample and some bone fragments from Barb's hipbone. He needed some time for the samples to dry and then to have a close look at them so Barbara and I went to McDonald's for a quick bite to eat. We returned to the clinic about forty minutes later and went back into the exam room. The dreaded word *leukemia* came out of his mouth as he began to describe what he saw under the microscope. He told us that 10 percent of the 30,000 white blood cells were immature. And that 35 percent to 40 percent inside the bone marrow were immature. This, he said, is the early sign of leukemia. He went on to say that this was not a death certificate and that it was very treatable. Even so, it was news that we both did not want to hear. All along I kept hoping that Barb had an infection of some kind that was causing the erratic white counts. We talked at length about some treatment schemes. We all agreed to start as soon as possible. After we left the clinic, we both broke down out in the parking lot. I can't begin to describe how devastated we both were at the time. We drove back to Carlisle and noticed that Barb's folks had arrived from Cape Cod. Since they were parked in our spot out front I pulled around back and we went in the back door. I went in first to try to break the bad news as easily as possible. It was a difficult task. Everyone was devastated by the news. I must say that this day was the worst in my life. I really felt bad when we first had the news about breast cancer, but this—after all we had been through in the past—was almost too much to take. We talked for a while then Barb decided that we needed to go out for dinner. We drove to Boiling Springs, Pennsylvania, to a local tavern, and had a great meal. Afterward, when we went back home, I told Barb that I didn't know if I could talk to our sons but I felt that I had to do it that night. Both were out at the time I called, but eventually called me back. I broke down with both of them. The emotions were just too high to hold back. They both passed on words of encouragement and said that we could get through this one more time. I also called her sister Sue, Jack O'Connor, our friend Jen Saltness, Donna Corbell, my sister Linda, and sister-in-laws Pam and Candy Domos. I asked Linda to call the rest of my family in Leavenworth and fill them in, since I was having such a difficult time.

To summarize the emotions, I guess you would say that sorrow was at the top of my list. Barbara did not deserve this, and I felt so helplessly sorrowful for her because I knew what she would have to go through again. Certainly, anger was present, but I was not clear about at whom it was directed.

The next morning Barb got up first and walked the dogs. I was exhausted and slept in until about 9:00 AM. She came in and said, "Come on you, get up. Let's start a new attitude today." Again there was that demonstration of a strong fighting spirit. She always said that I was her strength, but it was then that I realized how strong a woman I married. Barb stayed home and her folks and mine went with me to play nine holes of golf. We came back in about three hours, had lunch and then the women went out shopping for a new wig. I went over to the Carlisle Clinic to gather some information. I wanted to be sure that we could use the civilian doctor and hospital. I met with Pat Henry, who was the CHAMPUS administrator and the hospital administrator. I was told that Carlisle Barracks's clinic did not classify as a hospital. We were in a noncatchment area, which meant that we were farther than forty miles from the nearest military hospital and that we could choose any civilian doctor or hospital that we preferred. I picked up a copy of the referral for civilian treatment and placed it in Barbara's medical records. We had a wonderful meal that night and everyone was beginning to feel a little better. During dinner Dr. Ramos from KU Med returned a call that I had place earlier. I filled him in on the details that I knew at the time. He suggested that I ask Dr. Smith to send the bone marrow slide to the Armed Forces Institute of Pathology for another report. He also said that we should request that Dr. Smith look at the chromosomes. He used the terms *cytopathology* and *cytogenetics*. Cytopathology is a subspecialty of pathology used to diagnose diseases such as cancer or inflammation by looking at cells under a microscope. Cytogenetics is the study of chromosomes and chromosome abnormalities. Dr. Ramos told me that the lab would be able to determine whether or not some of Barbara's chromosomes had changed. He added that this information would be helpful to Dr. Smith in determining what kind of treatment he should prescribe for Barb.

My parents decided to leave early and have Barb's folks take them to the airport on Friday instead on Monday since Barb was going in the hospital on Monday. They offered to have my mother stay with me during the treatment, but I told them I would be OK and make the adjustment. That afternoon we all went to lunch and then we played a round of miniature golf. We had another wonderful meal that night and sat around and talked. Everyone offered whatever support could be provided. I was grateful that both of our sets of parents were with us during this difficult time. I know that it helped Barbara tremendously.

On June 24 Barb got a call from my sister Linda at about 9:00 AM. It was good that people were now getting over the initial shock and beginning to call and talk things out with Barbara. We had an appointment with Dr. Smith at 12:30 PM and one with Dr. Peter, the surgeon who would put in another Hickman, at 1:45 PM. At Dr. Smith's clinic they took another blood sample. The WBC was 31,900, and the platelets were 56,000. Not too much of a change from the Monday and Tuesday readings. We went into a small room off the main lobby to discuss the treatment procedures. Barbara asked most of the questions this time. She asked the doctor about the type of treatment he would prescribe and what he expected the outcome to be. She also asked about her chances of beating cancer again, since she had already fought off breast cancer. Her questions were direct and to the point and the doctor answered as honestly as he could. I told Dr. Smith about my conversation with Dr. Ramos and I requested him to send the bone marrow smear to the Armed Forces Institute of Pathology. I also mentioned the information about looking at the chromosomes.

When we got back home that evening, I figured the best way to inform all of our family and friends about the new cancer was to develop a form letter. Here is the letter that I wrote:

June 25, 1994

Dear Relatives and Friends:

I thought that it would be very useful to send this out to describe what is going on with our latest battle with cancer. We need your support and continued prayers; but Barbara will get through this, and I will be right there by her side pushing her along.

As you all know Barbara's last checkup in April at KU Med, was a good one. So this new cancer has just cropped up very quickly. One thing that I think you should all be aware of is that even though her last CAT and bone scan came up clear, it still would not have detected microscopic cancer cells lingering about. We have always known this, and generally looked for other signs that the breast cancer was kicking up again. But, when we left Leavenworth on the twelfth of April, Barb was in very good health with good counts on her blood samples. Since then we made the transition to life in Carlisle, and generally have been having a very good time.

About two weeks ago, Barbara began to notice that she was bruising very easily. I did not make the connection at the time. But it was time for her to go in for a checkup, so she made an appointment. She saw an OB/GYN doctor at the Carlisle Clinic. She asked him to take a blood sample. The sample showed that her white counts were out of whack and he said that she needed to see a specialist. Well, the short of all this is that we went to Dr. Smith who is a board certified in internal medicine, hematology and medical oncology, and he discovered through a bone marrow sampling that Barbara has the early stages of leukemia. After consultation, Barbara and I gained great confidence in Dr. Smith and his ability to treat and cure this disease.

I am going to list some definitions here so what I say about the treatment procedures may be a little clearer.

WBC—White blood count (Normal range for a woman: 4,800 to 10,800).

[blood] Platelets—One of the minute bodies found in the blood of higher vertebrates, essential to coagulation. (Normal range: 130,000 to 400,000)

Acute—violent, quickly (opposed to chronic, which is prolonged or lingering)

Myelogenous—*Meylo* is Greek for marrow, meaning spinal cord or bone marrow. *Genous* means generating, yielding, or produced by.

Leukemia—A generally fatal disease of the blood and blood-making tissues, characterized by a marked increase in the number of leukocytes, accompanied by anemia, exhaustion, etc.

Leukocyte—White or colorless blood corpuscle constituting an important agent in the protection against infectious diseases.

Marrow—A soft, vascular tissue found in the central cavities of bones.

Barbara was diagnosed with acute myelogenous leukemia. On Tuesday, June 21, Barbara's WBC was 33,000 and the platelets were 60,000. On Friday, June 24, her WBC was 31,900 and the platelets were 56,000. She will be hospitalized on Monday, June 27, 1994, to begin induction therapy.

Induction therapy means that for about seven days she will receive continuous chemotherapy. The goal is to get the bone marrow down to as near zero production of blood cells as possible. On day twelve another bone marrow sample will be drawn to see the results. If she is in remission at that point, then nothing else except recovery will begin. If not in remission, then they will repeat the chemotherapy. The whole process should take about four weeks in the hospital. She has to be in a controlled environment because she could develop an infection and will have no white cells to fight it off. Therefore, antibiotics are already prescribed to take care of the infection. At the end of the induction therapy, she should be in remission. By the way, I should point out here that her doctor said from the beginning that she is in the very early stages of leukemia, and that her type is: 1. not related to the breast cancer, and 2. it is very treatable, and he expects to cure her from leukemia. Her age and general physical health are excellent. So there is positive news in all of this.

At the end of the induction therapy, if in full remission, the doctor wants to do a bone marrow sample from her sister, Sue, to see if they match. The odds are one-in-four, but we are hopeful. If Sue is an exact match, we will proceed with a bone marrow transplant. There are a few options here. We can go to the military facility at Scott Air force Base in San Antonio, Texas, or we can choose a civilian treatment facility approved by the office in San Antonio. We have checked the local area, and several people, including her doctor have referred us to Johns Hopkins in Baltimore, Maryland. But for now that is a ways off. If Sue is not a perfect match, then we go to what is called consolidation therapy.

Consolidation therapy is the same treatment that I described above, only it is conducted two more times. The doctor would release Barbara between treatments to fully recover (about a month to six weeks), so that one treatment could drag out for a while. Again it is a full month of treatment and recovery in the hospital. In the event that this is the course that we have to take, and she has a relapse within the next year, then we move to the next course of action called nonrelated donor, bone marrow transplant.

Nonrelated means that we would go into the computer for the national bone marrow transplant center and check for a match from a donor. The odds of success are not as good as having a sibling as a donor even if we do find a match. There are a lot of things like DNA and chromosomes that are involved to get a perfect match.

A last but still experimental type of treatment is known as purging. Barbara's own marrow would be removed, purged, and placed back in her bones.

The big danger in all of this is during the first two years after treatment. The doctor said that if she stays in remission after the second year the success rate and survivability rate dramatically increases. He also feels that if we can get the bone marrow transplant it will in effect help fight off not only the leukemia, but the breast cancer as well.

I know that you are deeply concerned. God does listen, and this thing is beatable. You know that Barbara did a wonderful job fighting off the breast cancer, and she will do equally well this time. We are committed to fight and with your help, love and continued support, we will get through this together.

All our love,

NOTE: In discussions with Dr. Smith he gave us the following general stats concerning the various types of treatment:

Induction therapy—Remission rate at end of first month is 80 percent. In 75 percent to 80 percent of the cases, if nothing else is done, then a relapse will occur within the year.

Consolidation therapy—A 30 percent to 35 percent chance of total remission.

Bone marrow transplant—This is the optimal method with a 50 percent chance of total remission. Dr. Smith went on to add that the best time for total remission is after the patient stays in remission for two years.

On Saturday evening, June 25, Barb turned to me on the couch and said; "You know that there is a very good chance that I won't make it through this?" I told her that I had had that thought daily. So we decided to talk about her wishes if she died. She started and said, "Of course you know that I want to be cremated?" I responded, "Where do you want me to put your ashes?" She just smiled at me and said, "Put them in a jar on the mantel. That way every time you walk by you will think of me." I told her that was the most morbid thing she ever said. After a little more discussion about where the ashes should go, she finally said, "When you and the boys are ready just go somewhere and spread them outside." Barbara added that she only wanted a memorial service conducted in Leavenworth. She asked that Father Charlie McGlinn conduct the service and she requested that no morbid music be played. She asked me to keep it upbeat, and to remember her in death as she was in life. Barbara told me to take her clothes, jewelry, and perfumes and give them to our female relatives. The whole conversation only lasted about thirty minutes, but it was information that I would later find to be valuable. We had talked so much about positive things and beating cancer over the past eighteen months that we really had avoided discussing death. That thought was one that I had just chosen not to bring up.

On Sunday evening, the day before our trip back to the hospital to begin the new treatment, Barbara was depressed but determined to fight. We got some phone calls that day from Jack and Ellen O'Connor, Sue Moeller, sister Sue, brother John, and Donna Corbell. They all made Barb feel much better, knowing that she had friends and family in support. Barb fixed a wonderful supper, we walked the dogs and talked some more and went to bed ready to face the next round of battle with cancer.

11

BACK IN THE HOSPITAL

On June 27, 1994, we got up at 6:30 AM. Barb took the dogs out for a walk and I got ready to go to the hospital. We arrived at the hospital around 8:15 AM and went to admissions. Soon after, we went up to the preoperative surgery clinic where she would be prepared for the emplacement of the Hickman once again. She went into the operating room around 12:30 PM. Barbara received some plate-lets, had the operation, and was taken to recovery room number 602. Everything went well with the Hickman insertion and the nurses soon started to come in and change her clothing and dressings. Dr. Smith came by and talked for a while. Then Dr. Smith's nurse, Deb, came in to administer the first of the series of the chemotherapy. She drew some blood to send to the lab to look at the chromo-somes as we had requested.

Drugs and fluids taken:

Plateletts	IV
Idamycin	IV
Cytosar-U	IV
Zofran	

When the first three days of treatment were completed, Barbara was progress-ing just as the doctors expected. The only complications were constipation. The doctor ordered a stool softener to see if it would help. Other than feeling drained with no energy, Barb was doing OK. She did ask for some Compazine and Benadryl to help ward off the nausea. I went to the hospital every day after work and usually got home around 7:30 PM. Each day I had to keep pushing myself. It was much harder than the first time. I didn't believe that it was denial at all, although I did have a tremendous amount of anger that this was all happening again. The feeling of anger was never focused. It was never directed against any-one in particular. I guess I just felt sorry for the both of us, and it made me mad that my wife had to put up another struggle against cancer. My only consolation at that point was prayer. I resolved that with God's help we would both make it through this.

By June 30 everything was progressing as prescribed. Barbara's general attitude was good. Her skin color still seemed pretty good. She did, however, complain about the food tasting awful. I don't think it was the chemotherapy that was affecting her taste buds so much this time as it was just lousy hospital food.

We brought in the month of July with a phone call to our son Tom to wish him a happy twenty-forth birthday. It was now the second day after Barb finished the chemotherapy treatment. She was a little nauseated but generally doing all right, all things being considered. Barb remained constipated, but the doctor gave her something to help things along. Her spirit seemed to be pretty good but her white blood cell count was steadily on the decline. It was now down to 2,780.

The next day I got up at 7:30 AM and walked the dogs. After a cup of coffee and breakfast, I cut the grass and trimmed around the shrubs. I did some laundry and left for the hospital around 2:00 PM. Barb looked real good on this Saturday and her spirits were very high. She did say that she had a really bad night with a fever and not too much sleep. The fever was treated with Tylenol. At 4 PM I left the hospital to get us a spaghetti dinner from the Olive Garden restaurant in Harrisburg, Pennsylvania. It was about ten miles away but the service was quick. I drank a glass of beer while waiting for our food to be prepared. I returned to the hospital and we ate our meal. Barb really enjoyed having some good food for a change after a week of hospital food, but she remained constipated. Because of the fever and possible infection, Barb started getting antibiotics. She also got a blood transfusion of two pints of whole blood type O negative. Her white cell count was now down to 1,900, and she had a constant fever. I left the hospital around 7:30 PM.

By now my routine was pretty much as described above. I tried to spend as much time as I could with Barbara in the hospital and Sunday's were no exception. I got up, walked the dogs, and cleaned up a little around the house. I left for the hospital around 2 PM. When I arrived at the hospital I noticed that Barbara looked white for the first time. This was an indication that her blood counts were continuing to fall, which is exactly what the doctors wanted to happen. The whole idea of this induction therapy is to get the bone marrow down to producing as little as possible. The doctor had visited earlier and said that Barb's progress was good. Barb informed me that after I left the night before, she had a strong bowel movement. Now everything she eats seemed to come out in diarrhea. She told the doctor, but the doctor wants her to stay cleaned out to avoid any internal infection carried by bacteria in the digestive system.

Jack Mountcastle, my boss at Carlisle Barracks and his wife Susan, visited Barbara. I asked them to put out the word that Barb's white cell count was now very low and she was susceptible to infections. I explained to them that the doctor requested no more visitors. I was still allowed to visit as long as I remained healthy. All of the nurses were now wearing surgical masks when they came into the room.

Barbara mentioned to me that the area around the Hickman was sore and still red. She remained loose with continuous diarrhea throughout the day. I ate a fish sandwich at the hospital. We watched a soccer match of the World Cup and then I left for home. She had a fever of 102 degrees at 4 PM. Her white cell count had fallen to 610.

The next day was July Fourth, and I had the day off. Barb called me around 10:00 AM. She was upset, and I asked her what was wrong. She told me that the Hickman was the source of the infection and that it had to come out. This was a disappointing thing for her because she virtually had no veins to put an IV into. But her doctor said that it was only a minor setback and it was nothing that she should be concerned about. I thought, "Easy for them to say since they don't have to go through all the grief."

By the time I got to the hospital, the surgeon had already arrived and removed the Hickman. Barb was still upset about it. She said that they didn't deaden the area because the shot would have hurt as much as just pulling it out. So that is what he did; he just pulled out the catheter. Barb said it hurt like hell. The doctor told her that they would schedule her sometime in a few days to have another Hickman put in on the other side, which was her left breast area where the first one was emplaced back in Kansas. The IV team arrived and after the third attempt, they got an IV started. Barb and I had a Fourth of July picnic in her room. I brought in a couple of little flags, put them in her water glass and then went over to Kentucky Fried Chicken and got us each a meal. We had fried chicken, baked beans, corn on the cob, mashed potatoes and gravy, and dinner rolls. It was a very good day, and Barb's attitude remained good in spite of another trauma with the catheter. I checked with the attending nurse and found that Barbara's white cell count was now down to 330. I left the hospital around 7:30 PM.

When I got back to the hospital the next night, Barb told me that the night nurse had let the IV run dry and it clogged up. The IV team was furious but they managed to get in another one in the first try. This was the second complaint that

Barb had made to me about the hospital. A few days before, she said that the nurse call light stayed on for a good thirty minutes and all she wanted was some ice. By now I was furious so I called the hospital administrator. I told her about the problems that we were having and I also mentioned that the room was not cleaned to standard and that the coffee shop girl was rude and it was also a dirty place. She was apologetic and made a personal visit to see Barbara. We also got the head of the contracted cleaning team to visit. Barb continued to get an abundance of cards from concerned family and friends. She was truly loved and cared for by many people.

On July 6 I left work to go change clothes and leave for the hospital. When I got home, Dana Robertson and his wife were in my front yard. Dana was a lieutenant colonel who worked for me in Leavenworth, and was now arriving at Carlisle as a student at the Army War College. Dana wanted to drop off a car before he and his family went on their vacation to New Hampshire. This made me a little late in getting to the hospital. I arrived at the hospital around 6:00 PM. I picked up a hamburger on the way and ate in the room. Barb said that she was really beginning to feel the effects of her white count coming down. She went into her bathroom to try to clean up but found herself dizzy and weak. She looked pretty good and her spirits remained high. Barbara informed me that the associates treating her added a new doctor to the team. His name was Tom Burns. He was a consultant in infectious diseases. When I checked with the attending nurse I found that the white cell count was now at 200, but the good news was that Barbara did not have a fever all day. I guess you can always find a little bit of good news each day if you search hard enough. I left around 7:45 PM and drove home in a blinding rain and thunderstorm.

The next day was one of those real hot and muggy days when the temperature is well into the 90s, and I was sure that the humidity was real close to 90 percent. I talked to Barb around noon while I was eating my lunch. This is kind of a routine that we had developed. Get up, walk the dogs, go to work, come home for lunch, walk the dogs, call Barb, go back to work, come home, walk the dogs, go to the hospital, come home, walk the dogs, eat supper, watch the news, walk the dogs, go to bed. Barb told me that the surgeon was there talking to her and said that he would put in another catheter late that day. By the time I got to the hospital that night, it was over. The IV nurse came in and cleaned her up. I noticed that Barbara was really getting a lot of bruises and cuts. I felt so sorry for her that she had to go through all of this again. But, if it was successful, then she would heal and the marks in most cases would go away. I thought that having a few scars left over from beating cancer was not a big price to pay.

That day was an especially rough day for me. Dr. Tilford, PhD, an associate at work, came into my office and told me that Colonel Jeff Davis, the War College school secretary, mentioned to him that he heard that I was considering a compassionate reassignment. I told Dr. Tilford that it was the first that I had heard of it. I called Colonel Davis and we put the rumor to rest. In our conversation, I mentioned that if we could get the bone marrow transplant that I would be gone and in Texas for over three months and that we would need to get someone to help run the Strategic Outreach Program that I was in charge of at Carlisle. He was concerned about the health of Barb and said that if I needed anything, to just ask. He went on to talk about his brother. His brother's wife died from leukemia. No great details, but it was enough to ruin my day. The thought of Barbara dying had been on my mind constantly. I had several friends that had lost the battle to leukemia. It just seemed that I didn't know of anyone who had beaten that terrible disease. I had a lot of hope and a lot of faith in Barbara's will to fight, but I just feared the worse all the time.

July 8 was a day that both Barbara and I anxiously awaited. It was the twelfth day of the treatment. On that day Dr. Smith would take another bone marrow sample to see if the immature white cells had been suppressed. I called Barb around 9:30 AM to try to give her a boost since the sample was to be drawn around 10:00 AM. Unfortunately, the doctor had already finished. He told Barb that he would have the sample results by Monday and for her not to worry about it over the weekend. I went to the hospital around 5:30. Barb looked pretty good, but I could tell she was tired. She told me that Dr. Smith also took out some chips from the bone to look at them, too. The withdrawal of the samples was again very painful. We talked and watched TV. In our conversation I made a dumb comment about the dogs really being a pain in the ass taking care of them, and it really upset Barb. I reassured her that I was taking good care of them. I just forgot how sensitive she was. I remembered doing the same thing the last time she had the treatment back in Kansas. I reminded myself to be very careful in what I said because she was under such a tremendous amount of pressure. I remembered how we always said that we should always keep a positive attitude; but it was almost impossible during those trying times.

I left the hospital around 7:30 PM. As I arrived at our quarters, I noticed that my grass was cut and raked into little piles. Bill Doll, my neighbor, had cut the grass and was in the process of picking it up. I got us both a couple of beers, and we talked for a while. It was a rewarding experience to have people who you have only known for a couple of months come to your aid in the middle of a needed time. After a couple more beers, I walked the dogs, watched the news, and went to bed for some much-needed rest.

The next day was a Saturday, but not one that would see me sleep late. The dogs stirred around 6:00 AM, but I ignored them till 7:30 AM. After their walk I watered the lawn, did our laundry, and then vacuumed the house. I went to the hospital around 2:30 PM. Barb looked pretty good that day. She told me that Dr. Smith came by and said that the bone marrow looked real good. It was clean with no signs of immature white cells present. That was very good news. We would know the rest of the story on Monday when he got the results from the bone chips he sent to the lab. When I arrived in her room, Barb was in the process of getting another blood transfusion. She received two more bags of blood. That made a total of four to date and also two bags of platelets. She would probably receive more as she began her recovery process. I helped her to take a quick bath and wash her hair. Her hair was beginning to fall out a little bit, but nothing real noticeable yet. Barb ate her supper, and we watched the World Cup soccer match between Brazil and the Netherlands. I left early and came home around 6:30 PM. Barbara's white blood count now was at 190.

When I woke up Sunday morning, I thanked the Lord for another day and thought that it was the beginning of another week and that the next day, Monday, would be the beginning of the third week of Barbara's stay in the hospital. That was the bad thought for the day, and the positive thought was that I knew that she was halfway through the first treatment. I took out the dogs around 7:30 AM. I spent a little time out in the yard picking up branches and leaves from the storm that blew through over night. I finished edging the lawn, folded up the laundry, and scrubbed the downstairs bathroom. After lunch I took a quick nap. I walked the dogs again and then went to the hospital around 2:15 PM.

When I got to her room, Barb said that she had a pretty good night with plenty of sleep. She looked real good and again her spirits were high. We watched some golf and the World Cup then I went to the Red Lobster to get us a shrimp dinner. That was always a special treat for her to get away from eating the lousy hospital food. Before leaving I checked with the attending nurse as I did every day to see the status of Barbara's white cell count. The count went up just a fraction to 270. I went home around 7:30 PM. On the way home I kept thinking about what news we would get concerning the bone chip sample that Dr. Smith had sent off to the lab. I know that we were both praying for a good report. I also thought about how bored Barbara was getting with the time spent in the hospital, but her spirits remained high and she always had a smile for me. I kept thinking about how much better it would get as she began to recover and really started feeling better.

At work the next morning I was really anxious to find out if Barbara had heard anything from Dr. Smith about the results of the bone chip sample that he had sent off for analysis. I called around 8:30 AM to see if Dr. Smith had been by to see her yet. The answer was no. I called again around 9:45 AM, and Barb said that the bone chip sample was clean. I was elated. That was the best news that we had been given in a very long time. Barbara began crying over the phone, but I felt that those were tears of relief and joy this time instead of sadness.

I got to the hospital around 5:30 PM. Barb looked pretty good. We both talked about how glad we were concerning the outcome of the bone chip test. I knew that all of this was trying on Barbara. She would like nothing more than to be out of the hospital and enjoying life. I tried to keep her spirits up, even though she was in essence fighting for her life. Our bond of love was very strong and we were holding up all right. I felt that I was over the angry stage at that point. I no longer found that I had that awful sickening feeling in my stomach at night and I was not crying as much as I did in the beginning. It is odd what faith does for you. I didn't know where I would be without it. I was sure that the Lord listened to my constant prayers, and I knew that in some cases he lent a helping hand and healed the sick. I kept thinking about all the little children in the world who also were fighting for their lives against cancer. If Barbara did not make it through this then at least we could always say that we had the blessing of the Lord to spend almost twenty-six wonderful years together. That is a lot to be thankful for, but very hard to accept because we wanted nothing more than many, many more years together.

12

BEGINNINGS OF A DOWNFALL

In my now daily ritual, I called Barb at noon after taking our dogs for a walk. She didn't sound very good on the phone. I asked her what was wrong, and she said that she had a temperature of 103 degrees the previous night. It broke with Tylenol, but this was the highest that she had ever had. We both felt that there was trouble with the new catheter. Since Barbara had such bad luck with the catheters, it just seemed that this new one was probably the source of the infection that was pushing her temperature so high. This would be another minor setback, but a painful one for Barb since she had trouble with the IVs in her arms. I hoped and prayed that the doctors could isolate the infection and correct it.

After work I walked the dogs and then took my Audi into the shop to get an overheating problem corrected. We were planning a big trip to Cape Cod in August when our sons arrived in Pennsylvania, and we needed the bigger car to transport us all. I picked up and turned in some shirts at the dry cleaners, looked at some portable CD players in the Post Exchange shopping center, and then left for the hospital.

I arrived around 5:15 PM. Barb was very upset and started to cry as soon as I walked in her room. Dr. Burns had visited her around 4:00 PM and was concerned with the high temperature. The nurses continued to break it with Tylenol, but the doctor wanted to get to the source of the infection that was causing it. He told Barb that he was putting her on a new antibiotic called amphotericin B that fought fungus. It was a strong drug and could cause some severe reactions. He did not want to wait for the results of the culture tests being run to determine the source of the infection. Barbara was scared and could only imagine the worst. I tried to reassure her that she was in good care and that they would be careful. She really had no option at this point. While I was at the hospital, Barb received another bag of platelets. I talked with the nurse to see how dangerous this new drug was. The nurse told me the most commonly observed infusion-related side effects of amphotericin B are fever, chills, and muscle pain. I felt reassured that things would be OK and Barb felt comfortable with it also after we talked. We simply could not allow her to continue to have high temperatures. Barb mentioned that her hair was starting to fall out in globs. I noticed that it looked dull and dry.

We received a phone call from Jack O'Connor and my mother to say hello and see how things were going. Barbara's white count remained low at 340, which was not helping her fight off the infection that appeared to be getting the best of her.

I continued in my daily routine and tried to get some things done at work, but it was difficult to apply any focus. All I could do was think about my wife and the horrible condition that we found ourselves in each day. The positive attitude was becoming real hard to maintain in spite of our vow to fight this cancer. I went to the Army shopping exchange after work and bought a Sony Walkman for Barb. I got to the hospital around 5:30 PM. Barbara really looked worn out. I could tell that the new antibiotic was taking its toll on her. The doctors reassured her that she would be fine in about a week. Her hair was really starting to fall out fast. Barb had an upset stomach and spit up just a little. When I left she said that she would be just fine. At home I had a call on our answering machine from a dear old friend, Evelyn Fish from Fort Worth, Texas. Then I received a call from one of my old fraternity brothers, Tim Theurer. I remained grateful for the outpouring of concern for both Barbara's health and mine. It was really hard for people to call because they didn't usually know what to say. They really wanted me to talk and tell them that everything was going to be all right. Unfortunately, there are no magic cures for cancer. I guess people were afraid when they heard the word *cancer* and rightfully so. I just tried to reassure anyone that called that Barbara was getting the best advice and treatment that she could and that she was a strong person who vowed to fight to the end.

All that night I kept thinking and praying for a change in our luck. I kept watching for signs that things would get better. Barbara was now taking potassium to supplement some chemical loss to her body. Her fever continued, and she had the nurses bringing her Tylenol every four hours to keep the temperature in check. Her hair was really falling out. It was just like the last time back in Kansas and was starting to get all over everything. I continued to clean her gown up and removed a lot of loose hair. That night was the worst that Barbara had ever felt in all her time in the hospital. I tried to comfort her, but with the fever, lack of sleep at night, and the constant worry that her final Hickman would clog, she was simply exhausted. She continued to cough a lot and spit up some phlegm on occasion. Her white cell count showed no great signs of improvement, remaining at 230. She was in the beginning stages of a losing battle with an infection. Her only hope was for her bone marrow to kick in and push out some good white cells to help the antibiotics fight off the yet unknown infection that was sapping the life out of her.

The next morning, July 15, I called Barb to see how her night went. She told me that her temperature rose to 104 degrees. The nurses were giving her Tylenol III, which contained codeine, to control the fever. I keep asking her what the doctors were saying. I could feel my helplessness and frustration. She said that they were concerned about the high temperatures but felt that the treatment was going as scheduled.

When I arrived at the hospital that night, I noticed that Barbara had brushed and pulled at her hair to get rid of the remaining globs. It was almost all gone by now. I spent some time cleaning her up. I also noticed that there was a lot of hair around the bed on the floor. I told the nurse to get someone from housekeeping to mop up the floor. I told Barbara that we were definitely not going to use this hospital again. Barb received a bag of platelets and then I drove back home got a Philly steak and cheese sandwich and drank a couple of beers and then went to bed.

I didn't wake up till 8:00 AM the next day, Saturday, July 16. I could feel the exhaustion in my body. The lack of sleep and constant worrying was taking its toll on my physical condition. After taking the dogs for a walk, I spent some time outside picking up some sticks that had blown into the yard with the previous night's thunderstorm. I watered and fertilized all of our plants and returned inside. While I did the laundry, I made some lunch and got ready to go to the hospital.

When I arrived at the hospital I could not see much change in Barbara's condition. She still looked tired and worn out. I tried to comfort her some by giving her a back rub. We talked and I tried to console her as best as I could. I knew that she was not in any pain, but I could tell that the length of the hospital stay was starting to get to her. I know that she was really beginning to lose patience, but she was just not healthy enough to be released. All that day I kept thinking how difficult it would be for her to return in six weeks to start the second treatment. She was definitely going to need a lot of love and encouragement to get her attitude back up to a fighting level. I stayed at the hospital with her till 6:30 that night, leaving early so I could get home to cut our grass before it got dark. After cutting the grass, I sat on my deck with my neighbor Bill Doll, drinking beer till 11:00 PM. It was a needed break.

Sunday morning arrived too soon, and I could feel the effects of too much beer the night before. I felt a little down when I got up and I felt the beginning of a sinus headache. I took some ibuprofen, ate breakfast, went to church, and came home and just relaxed. I knew that I really had to go to the store to get some food but I just felt lousy. I lay around most of the day trying to get rid of the headache.

Around 6:00 PM. I felt a little better so I left for the hospital. Barb looked real tired. In fact she kept taking little catnaps while I was there. She also had a hot water bottle going on her side, where she said that she was real sore. The doctor ordered an X-ray, but we had no word as to the results. We both agreed that the doctors wanted to make sure that Barbara's kidneys were OK. After checking with the head nurse I found out that Barbara's white cell count was only 280. I left the hospital around 7:30 PM still feeling the effects of the sinus headache.

At home that night I received a call from Donna Corbell, a dear friend from Texas. She wanted to know how everything was going with the treatment and to see if it was all right for her to call Barb. I told her that Barbara would love to hear from her. I took some more medicine and went to bed around 9:00 PM.

When I got up the next day the sinus headache wasn't much better. I got ready for work and called Barbara as soon as I got to my office. She told me that the results of the X-ray revealed that she had a slight case of pneumonia. This was not a blow, or a setback; it just caused Barbara more discomfort. I continued to suffer from the sinus headache. At 4:00 I finally went to the medical clinic to see a doctor. He put me on some stronger antibiotics to help clear up the sinus and ear infection. Because of the infection and me feeling so lousy I decided to not go to the hospital. I talked to Barb several times on the phone. She said that she had a fairly good night and did manage to get a little sleep. She also said that she received platelets the night before, but the nurse failed to administer a drug beforehand to help ward off a reaction. Barb got the chills and threw up. She said that it was awful but that she was OK. My son Tom called me to check up on his mother. We had a good long talk then I watched a little TV and went to bed. I really felt sick and guilty because I couldn't go to the hospital.

The next morning I called Barb from work. She said that Dr. Smith had visited and told her that her bone marrow was producing a lot of good cells. He told her that he felt her progress was good. He also changed his mind about the treatment schedule. He said that he wanted to go forward with a search for a donor and go immediately into a bone marrow transplant instead of a second session of chemotherapy. I hadn't talked to him yet but I wanted to find out why he was changing the game plan. Dr. Smith also told Barb that he felt that she could be released from the hospital on Friday or Saturday providing her white count was sufficient. Barbara was pleased with that news. She was more than ready to come out of the hospital and rest up at home.

With the news of an eminent release, Barb told me to check out the location of the Wigwam store in Camp Hill, Pennsylvania. She wanted to go directly from the hospital to the shop and get a new wig. That day I did not go to the hospital because I wanted the antibiotics that I was taking to succeed. I simply did not want to put Barbara in any jeopardy at all, and I knew that I had a slight infection. I did more or less the same thing that I did the day before after work. I just rested at home and let the drugs do their work. I got rid of the headache almost immediately after taking the first decongestion pill. Boy was it ever a relief to feel halfway human again.

I called Barbara from home that evening and talked to her for a long time. I kept telling her how bad I felt because I couldn't go to the hospital to visit. She told me that I had to take care of myself and not to worry about her, that she was being well taken care of by the nurses. I had her check with the head nurse and found out her white blood count was only 140. This was really a mystery to me as to why her count was not rising faster.

On July 20 I felt a lot better and thought it was safe enough to go to the hospital. When I arrived I put a surgical mask on just to be sure that I was not spreading any germs. Barbara did not look good at all. I could really see that all of this illness was a physical toll on her body. I knew in my heart that she could recover over time, but at time I felt so sorry that such a beautiful woman had to suffer all of these indignities again. I also noticed that she was a lot more irritable than ever before. I just prayed that it was not a sign of desperation or despair. She had done so well up to that point. Most of her hair had fallen out except some fuzzy stuff in front and in the back. She asked me to bring her a pair of little blue scissors on my next visit to trim up the remaining puffs of hair. Barbara was still running high fevers. She got nauseated twice while I was there and spit up. I noticed that there was blood in the spit. There was not a lot of blood, but enough that I felt I should ask her about it. When I mentioned it, she became very upset, but admitted that blood had been present in her spit for the past couple of days. I stayed until 8:00 PM and then left. I checked with the head nurse before I left and she told me that the white count was 140 and that they were going to give Barbara another bag of platelets after I left. I drove back home through Camp Hill to find the Wigwam so we wouldn't have to hunt for it when Barbara got released from the hospital.

The next night after work I planned to cut the grass before going to the hospital, but it rained. I arrived at the hospital around 5:30 PM. Barbara still looked sick, and she felt miserable. She told me that she had been throwing up all day and she continued to do so while I was there. I was really starting to get concerned about her pneumonia. I kept thinking that the doctors needed to change the antibiotics; it was obvious to me that the ones that they were giving her were not helping. In all of her misery, I tried my best to comfort her as much as possible, but I could see that nothing was going to ease her discomfort. Barbara looked tired, so I told her to get some rest while I monitored the IV machines. She took a nap for about twenty minutes, and I could tell that she really slept hard. Just before I left she had a fever of 103 degrees, and her white count was still very low at 170.

All the way home and for the rest of that night, I prayed real hard for just a little break. I felt that she so deserved a chance to recover and come home for a rest. I kept telling myself that everything was going to be fine and as soon as she was strong enough that the doctors would let her come home.

The next morning at work I called Barbara to see if she was feeling any better. She told me that she managed to keep some of her breakfast down. She also said that the doctors took a sample of her throw up for lab analysis. The really bad news was that at that early hour she already had a fever of 104 degrees.

All throughout that day at work I kept thinking that I should leave and go to the hospital to try to lend a hand. I didn't know why, but I just felt better if I were at her side. I did finally leave and got to the hospital a little earlier than usual. Barbara's condition was about the same. She was really sick with the pneumonia and the high fevers. The whole time during this visit all she did was cough and spit up. I kept her mouth wiped off and constantly rinsed out the emesis basin. My mother called to check on Barbara but Barb quickly handed me the phone. She was just too sick to talk to anyone. I felt a deep sense of depression creeping into our lives. Was this what it was all going to come down to after such a long hard fight? I was really struggling with my faith. I kept reassuring Barbara that the pneumonia would start to break up and that she would feel a lot better soon. But whom was I really trying to convince that things would work out? I was scared, both for me and for Barbara. I had never seen a person this sick before, and to see my best friend and spouse so ill was tearing my heart out.

The only good news that I was able to get that day was that her white count was starting to come up. Barbara's white cell count rose to 320, but she was still in great danger. I kept hoping and praying that she could build up enough immunity to help in the fight. I left the hospital that night with a lot of mixed emotions.

When I got up the next morning I found that the emotional confusion continued. I sat at the breakfast table drinking a cup of tea and started to cry. It was a well-deserved cry and the beginning of an emotional release. I was a very sad man. When I finished my cry I felt better. I had a new resolve. I had regained some strength that I knew I would need to help her through the fight with cancer.

I got back to the hospital around 1:00 PM. Barbara looked worse than when I left her the night before. She had lost all of her strength. Her eyes were blood red from a lack of platelets, and bruises surrounded them. She was also now receiving oxygen through a little butterfly tube in her nose. I kept thinking that my new resolve may have been in vain. But I mustered the strength to try to help her out. I kept a cold washcloth on her head most of the day and just talked to her in an encouraging voice.

Barbara slept most of the day, which she badly needed. All I could do was be there for her and provide as much comfort as possible.

All day long I kept replaying the scenario of her death. In some small way I knew that if she did die that she would be so much better off than living a life constantly fighting cancer. I prayed constantly for this not to happen. I asked God for a little break to give her a chance of recovery. I knew in my heart that if she could get over the pneumonia then there was no doubt that she could beat the cancer once again. I went over all of the joy that we had enjoyed in our life. But all I could do was cry when I looked at her in her current condition. The scenario of her death plagued my mind. I hated the thought of telling her sons. But I vowed that if that time came then I would try my best to fulfill her wish of honoring her in death as we had in life. I kept thinking over and over again how hard it all would be, and the only consolation that I got was the thought that she would be at peace and not fighting cancer.

That night at home I was really depressed. I talked to my mother and told her I didn't know if Barbara would make it. She was concerned and tried to offer me some encouragement. I just had a sick feeling in my stomach that she was too sick to survive.

I did not sleep well that night. I kept waking up at odd hours and immediately began praying for a little break. I told God that a miracle would be nice, but if he was not in the miracle granting business then just a little break to help Barbara along.

I finally slept a little and got up around 7:30 AM. I walked the dogs, got something to eat, and then got ready for church. It was kind of odd that the Gospel that day was about Jesus performing the miracle with the bread and fish. It reassured me that if God did want a miracle then it was still possible, even under the most severe circumstances.

As I drove over to the hospital all I could think about was the terrible condition that my wife was in. When I approached the elevator I took a deep breath and said one last prayer for a little break. As I walked down the hall toward Barbara's room I saw one of the attending nurses, Anna. She looked at me and said, "A little better today." I asked about the white count and she told me that it had improved to 400. For that brief moment I knew that the Lord had answered my prayers.

Throughout the rest of the day I could see positive signs of improvement in Barbara's condition. The coughing was less severe and she was perspiring a lot, which meant that the fever was breaking. Her temperature did rise every so often but it was not nearly as bad as the few previous days. Barbara drifted in and out of sleep most of the day, but I knew that she needed it real bad. I managed to get her to eat a few bites of her lunch and we talked a little. I kept her forehead wiped down with a cool washcloth and helped her to the bathroom when needed. The attending physician stopped by and told me that they were working on an oral antibiotic that Barbara could take at home after her release. I couldn't help but think that this was the break that she needed so badly. Things were so much improved from the previous day. I left the hospital with a much better attitude and a great deal of hope that my beloved was on her way to recovery. I wrote in my journal "Great day."

When I returned to the hospital the next night I soon realized that the entry the night before in my journal was not exactly the right phrase. Because of the little progress that I witnessed the day before, I really thought Barbara was on the road to recovery. But this muggy Monday night at the end of July did not present a scene of recovery; rather one of despair and more heartache.

Barbara's condition was nowhere near what it had been the day before. She was hot with fever and talking out of her head in a completely delirious state. I couldn't explain it so I simply believed that it was all a result of the high fevers. She was really a mess. She didn't want to eat even though she remained very weak. I left the room and went out to the parking garage before I turned around and went to the hospital snack bar. I bought a small fruit bowl and took it back to her room. I was convinced that she was not eating properly and the least that I could do would be to get her to at least eat some fruit. I took the fruit back to her room and fought with her to eat a little. She was so sick and angry that I was trying to make her eat. She eventually pushed my hand away and said very angrily, "That's enough!" I finally left the hospital.

I realized that Barbara was not getting any better and I felt that nourishment had a great deal to do with her gaining back some strength. I decided to take the next day off and be at the hospital with her as long as I could. My goal was to be there when the meals were delivered so I could see that she at least ate a little.

I got up the next morning at 6:00 AM and arrived at the hospital by 7:00. Barbara was awake and surprised to see me. When she spoke it was with a slur like someone drunk. I could see right away that there was no change in her condition. I looked at her chart to see what the temperature recordings were throughout the night. The highest was 100 degrees.

When the breakfast arrived I got her to eat a few bites. She would ask me for her water or juice, and I would hold it up to her mouth. This seemed to irritate her and she took the glass away from me, but failed to drink. I told her to drink her water but she only responded that she already had finished. I had to work real hard throughout the day just to get any kind of nourishment in her. Her weakened condition had also prompted the nursing staff to put a bedside port-a-potty in her room so she didn't have to try to make it all the way to the bathroom. Even getting out of bed to sit on the potty became a major operation. We worked out a routine where she would roll her legs over the side of the bed while I lifted her up. Then by turning to avoid tangling up the IV lines, we would swing around together till she was properly seated.

Throughout the rest of the day Barbara remained delirious. She talked almost constantly and at random, not making much sense at all. At one point I said, "Barbara, where are you?" She said that she was in her bedroom at Leavenworth and that a man was trying to sell her a house for $160,000, but I wouldn't let her buy it. The odd part of it all was that she was actually carrying on the conversation with the mystical man in her bedroom in Leavenworth. I would say that about 99 percent of the day she was off in another world. She told me that she was in Lansing, in her waterbed. She also asked several times where the "kids" were. I knew that she was referring to our two sons, but they were grown men. At one point she told me, "Isn't this the shits, only two months ago I was the president of the United States, now it will be very hard to go on."

I tried to figure out what was wrong with her and why she remained in a delirious state. The only thing that I could figure was causing all of this was the many days of high fever that was making her talk out of her head. This was the most confusing day for me ever. When Barbara wanted something she asked for

Kleenex or water in a coherent voice. But by the time I handed it to her she was back in la la land and talking out of her head again.

By mid-afternoon Dr. Williams, one of the attending oncologists came by to check on Barbara. I voiced my concerns about Barbara's condition. She could only respond that everything depended on the bone marrow's ability to produce good white cells to help fight off the infection.

Barbara continued to lie there on the hospital bed in the same delirious condition throughout the rest of the day. At one point she spoke out when she saw a horse on the TV. She said, "Joe Stone, his roommate. He races with the stones, Army stones. You know tuna bread and stuff like that." I was so distraught that I cried. I couldn't do a thing to help her, and I did not know what was wrong. To keep my mind off of the events, I wrote in my journal and tried to comfort her as much as I could. At one point she saw a courtroom scene on the TV and started talking like she was the prosecuting attorney.

I stayed at the hospital till 9:00 PM and decided that she was resting enough so that I could go get some sleep. Little did I know at that time that the worst was yet to come.

13

PULMONARY ARREST & ICU

On July 27 I arrived at the hospital around 7:45 AM. I checked the hospital chart and found that Barbara did not have a fever the previous night. She did remain delirious and continued to talk out of her head. She seemed distressed and had difficult time breathing, but insisted that she was in no pain. She was restless and moved about quite a bit. I did manage to get her to eat a few bites of cold cereal and drink some orange juice.

The attending nurse and a nurse trainee came into the room to change the bedding and wash Barbara. I assisted as much as possible. Barbara was really hard to handle at this point because of her listless state and no strength. We managed to get her on the bedside commode and then the nurses proceeded to wash her all over. They gave her a Darvocet to help relax her just a little. I rubbed her feet, and she drifted off to sleep. It was the first time that I saw her really resting peacefully in a long time.

Dr. Williams came by to examine Barbara. I told her that she was tired and asked her not to wake her. I asked the doctor what the planned course of action was at this point. She explained that if Barbara's white count rose naturally, then we would continue on course. If her white count rose slowly, then they would continue to treat with the antibiotics to fight the infection and wait and see what the progress would be. If the white count was not coming up because of the leukemia still affecting the bone marrow, then they would consider more chemotherapy to kill it off. I told her that Barbara could not take any more chemotherapy, that it would kill her. She did not disagree. The doctor noticed that Barbara's blood pressure was starting to drop and she ordered the nurses to increase the fluids in the IVs. Her final comment to me before she departed was, "I've had patients sicker than this, and they still recovered."

About five minutes after the doctor left, Barbara said to me, "Tommy, I've got to pooh." Since there was no one else around I did my best to get her out of the bed and on to the bedside commode. I noticed that she had diarrhea and had already started to go. After I got her on the pot I walked around the bed to ring the nurses' bell to get someone to come in and help me clean up the mess. When no one came right away I stepped out in the hall to look for a nurse. I came back to Barbara's aid at the pot and asked her if she was all right. She groaned at me, in a drowsy state, and her head slumped to one side. I went back out in the hall and found a nurse and told her that I needed some help. When I returned to the room I noticed that Barbara had gone limp. I put my ear up to her mouth and could only hear a very faint sound of breathing. The nurse arrived, and I told her that I didn't think that Barbara was breathing. At that point Barbara took a couple of gasps for air and stopped breathing.

The emergency call went out from the nurse, and the room immediately filled with fifteen to twenty people. They grabbed Barbara and threw her on the bed stripping her gown and began mouth-to-mouth resuscitation. An attending medic arrived within seconds and jammed an artificial breathing apparatus down her throat. One of the nurses turned to me and suggested that I should leave. She said, "It is going to get pretty ugly."

I told her that I was all right.

She continued with, "You look a little white."

I wanted to respond, "What the hell do you think I should look like?" But I kept my head and told her that if I needed to leave the room, then I would.

I stood in the room and watched the horrible event unfold. I watched as Barbara's color turned to a purple-black. The head cardiologist stood in the middle of the attending team. He was in complete control of the entire operation. He closely watched the monitors and commanded when to start and stop the artificial respiration. After several tense minutes and one milligram of epinephrine and atropine, I heard one of the technicians cry out, "I have a pulse!" I was too much in shock to get any joy out of her comment. In my heart I knew that I had just held my wife while she gasped her last breath.

The team continued to work on Barbara trying to get her blood pressure stabilized. At that point Dr. Williams and I had a quick conversation about options for further treatment. I told her that I wanted Barbara to have the best care possible and to give her every chance for a recovery.

While we were talking the nurses wheeled Barbara out of the room and took her up on the elevator to the intensive care unit (ICU). The doctors and nurses huddled around me to offer some comfort. I kept telling them that I was OK and that I wanted to go up to the ICU. When I got to the ICU, the doctors and nurses were in the room hooking Barbara up to a variety of IV injections and the respirator. Dr. Williams told me that Barbara had had a pulmonary arrest, which meant that she stopped breathing, and it was not a heart attack. She explained that this was common for patients in Barbara's condition, and that they would know more about her condition after they got her stabilized.

I sat in the ICU room while the doctors continued their work. I tried my best to keep my mind busy and off of the tragedy that I had just witnessed. I kept thinking that I had just watched Barbara die, and it would only be a matter of time until one of the doctors said that she was finally gone. The one thing that I did do was make sure that all of the attending staff knew that I did not want Barbara kept alive by any mechanical process. I also requested that the hospital staff contact a priest to administer Barbara her last rites.

After several minutes of listening to the respirator and looking at all of the tubes poked into my wife's body, I had to leave the room. I took my chair just outside the door. I just couldn't stand it to be there at that point, waiting for her to finally pass on to the Lord.

Soon Father Havalon, from a parish in Harrisburg, Pennsylvania, arrived at the hospital. I spoke briefly with him, and then he went into the room to pray and administer last rites. I could not bring myself to go in with him, but I could hear as he said the words of prayer over Barbara. I cried a lot in pain and sorrow. When the priest came out of the room, we took a short walk down the corridor. I questioned him about the Church's position on cremation. He told me that the Church honored cremation, but the ashes had to be buried. I asked him if I could leave her remains in Harrisburg and go to Leavenworth for a memorial service, and he assured me that it was all right. I really had to do some soul searching now because Barbara's wishes were for her ashes to be spread, not buried.

After the priest left, I sat alone outside of the room. I was convinced that Barbara's spirit was no longer in her body. All that remained of her was a swollen corpse in a hospital ICU room. I thought that if she were to survive all of this then God would have had to send her spirit back to rejoin her body.

With each passing moment my anxiety rose. I finally changed my mind about sitting in the room, and I moved my chair back by her bedside. It was extremely hard to sit in the room listening to the hum of the machines, and I found myself staring at the monitor waiting for the wave lines to go flat. At this time Barbara's heart was racing quickly. Her heart rate was 155 with a blood pressure of 83/47. The doctors explained that they were most concerned about the blood pressure and were using drugs to keep it up until her body could do it on its own.

Around 2:00 PM I took a walk back to room 602 where Barbara had lived the final days of her life. The nurses had packed up all of her personal belongings. I gathered them up and took them out to my car. I walked around the parking lot, had a long and hard cry, and then went back to the hospital. I went into the snack bar, had a cup of coffee and a piece of pie, and then returned to the ICU around 3:00 PM.

The work by the doctors was pretty much the same as it had been. They were using the ventilator tube to help suction out Barbara's lungs. The dopamine was continued to keep her blood pressure up. Her heart rate was steadily decreasing and now registered at 142 beats per minute. I decided that I needed to make some phone calls to inform the family members. Before I left the ICU ward I had Dr. Smith give me the clinical diagnosis. He said that Barbara was comatose and not expected to live.

I went down to the hospital administrator's office and told her that I needed access to a phone with some privacy. They escorted me to an empty office. I made several attempts to contact my sons, parents, and Barbara's parents. No one was home and I felt it inappropriate to leave such a distressful message on answering machines. I returned to the ICU ward and talked some more with the doctors. They told me that they would not know anything for the next twelve to twenty-four hours. In essence, it was out of their hands at that point. I stayed at the hospital till around 6:00 PM and then returned to my home. I had to get on the phone to notify my family, rest a little, and get something to eat.

I placed all the calls again and still got no response. This time, however, I left messages to have my call returned. The first one to call me back was my younger brother, Steve. We talked for a short while and he said, "You need some help." He told me that he would make arrangements for the next flight out of Kansas City. The next person to call back was my son Tom. He was angry and wanted to come right away. I told him that I didn't know if his mother would still be alive when he got there and that I would not take him to the mortuary to view her if she were dead. He said that he didn't care and he wanted to leave right away. I told him that I would check on the flight arrangements and call him back. In the meantime, my son Jason called. He had been out with a few friends and his roommates had gone and found him. Jason was also angry and hurt. He told me that he did not want to see his mother in a comatose condition. I told him that I understood his feelings and that I would call him back after I had made some flight arrangements.

It is difficult to explain what I was going through at that moment. I was alone, in shock, hurting badly and yet I had to keep my wits long enough to do the informing and make travel arrangements. It was the most horrible night in my entire life. After several hours on the phone talking to the rest of our family members and the airlines, I was exhausted and needed some sleep. I called the hospital at 11:57 PM to check on Barbara's condition. The attending nurse said that she was stable with a heart rate of 130, blood pressure of 80/50 and a temperature of 101 degrees. She also informed me that the white cell count rose to 300 and that Barbara was a little less responsive to touch. Needless to say I had a restless night.

The next morning I finally got out of bed around 7:00 and took the dogs for their morning ritual. I felt compelled to clean the house up a little because I knew that Barbara would not like her sons to see her home in a mess.

I arrived at the hospital around 11:40 AM. Barbara's general condition was about the same. I did notice however that she opened her eyes for the first time. The attending nurses kept a close watch on all of the instruments and constantly suctioned out the brown nasty fluid from her lungs. I leaned over my dear wife and tried to talk to her in a very gentle way. I told her that her two sons were on their way to see her. It was most disheartening not getting any kind of a response, but I resolved that I would continue to talk to her in the hopes that she could at least hear. At that point I made the biggest decision in my life. I started to cry, but I held her hand tightly and leaned over close to her ear. I told her that I loved her very much and that if she had the will and the power to die because she was tired of fighting, then I would never hold it against her.

Of course, I received no response. But I knew that both of us had vowed a long time before to fight to the end. I guess in essence I was telling her it was OK for her to give up. I knew that it was contrary to her will, but I just hated seeing her in such a condition with the possibility of many more years of fighting for her life. She had always been such a vibrant woman full of life and love and now she had lost it all. I also remember thinking at the time that she was not really alive because her spirit had left the body. At that point I had absolutely no hope of her ever recovering.

I took a seat in the ICU room by Barbara's bed. It was a place that I would occupy for many hours. I kept staring at the monitor and saying to myself, "You are doing what you said you wouldn't do," and that was just sitting there waiting for her to die once more. It was sheer torture.

The nurses kept coming in and forcing Barbara to cough through the tube so they could suction more lung fluid. They also withdrew some of her stomach fluid, which contained the nutrients from the tube feeding. They told me that the amount indicated that her stomach was not absorbing the feeding. I left the room to go get a cup of coffee.

When I returned I found myself going through a lot of different thoughts. Just a few hours before, I was firmly convinced that there was no life in the body on the bed. Now I was not sure. I knew that her heart was beating on its own, and that she was breathing as well. I guess when I saw her open her eyes I changed my mind. Her stare was not focused, but never the less she did it on her own. At that point I found myself talking to her a lot more. I told her that she was strong and doing a great job. I had reverted back to the positive attitude that we had both practiced. It didn't seem strange like crying and hanging on to a dying loved one at all. Rather it was natural and comforting. I just tried to reassure her and talk to her in a normal voice without a lot of emotion.

I walked down the hall looking for my two brothers who were due to arrive around 2:00 PM. At 2:30 PM they had not arrived, and I had to leave for the airport to pick up my two sons.

As soon as both of my sons came off the plane we hugged and cried. It was difficult. I tried to find the strength for them to hold them up and to try to make it through all the grief together. When we got to the hospital, Jason decided that he did not want to see his mother. I told him that it was all right and that it was a decision that he had to make. I sat my oldest son down and explained to him exactly what he would see when he went into the room. I knew that he had never seen someone critically ill, let alone his mother. We walked into the room and he was really great. He spent a considerable amount of time with his mother just talking to her and holding her hand. He was a lot stronger than I knew. My two brothers arrived shortly after Tom and I were back in the room. My brother Steve went to the waiting room to be with Jason. I felt comforted knowing that I finally had some of my family with me to help out.

After several hours in the ICU room, we all decided that it was time to go. I stopped and picked up a big bottle of wine for dinner. That night we started a toasting ritual to Barbara and an increase in her white blood cell count. It seemed to give us something to focus on for the time being. It was really great having my sons there. We sat up until late that night and discussed all the possibilities. I told them of their mother's wishes and the arrangements that would have to be made if she passed away. Both of them were good and understanding, but still hopeful for a recovery. I was not as optimistic.

I got up the next morning at 7:10 with the dogs. I came back and tried to get some more rest but was unable to go to sleep. At 8:30 I called the ICU ward to check on Barbara's status. The attending nurse told me that Dr. Williams had been in the hospital and tried to call me. I asked her what number she had dialed and found out that they had the wrong phone number on Barbara's chart. I was furious and told them to get it straightened out. In the meantime she patched me through to the doctor. Dr. Williams told me that Barbara's general condition was about the same. She did have a little fever during the night but the nurses were able to bring it down. The doctor went on to explain that she got a pupil response from Barbara during the morning exam. I asked her if this was an involuntary reflex. She said only the brain can make the pupils constrict. This indicated that there was evidence of at least some brain activity. Dr. Williams also told me that Barbara's white cell count jumped to 800. I was startled and thought, "Maybe the wine toast was a good idea." The doctor told me that the plan for the day was to conduct a CAT scan of the brain to check for any bleeding or masses. She also wanted to try some more tube feeding by thinning down the liquid to see if the stomach could absorb it. I asked her why she didn't just feed her nourishment through the IVs, and she said that it was too risky because of the richness of the IV fluids and the possibility of bacteria and more infection.

After we hung up I kept going over everything that I had seen the day before. I couldn't get the thought out of my head that Dr. Williams had said that Barbara's condition was "poor but not impossible." I had told her that her statement was a double negative and I preferred to interpret it as "poor, but possible." Maybe there was some hope after all.

My son Tom and I got to the hospital around 11:25 AM. The technicians were just taking Barbara out for the brain scan. We had a quick visit and I told Barbara what her white count was and what they were going to do with her for the day. The nurse told me that she would be gone for about forty-five minutes, so Tom and I went to the snack bar.

At 12:40 we went back up to the ICU. Barbara was being rolled back toward her room. For the first time I saw both of her eyes open. Soon Tom and I returned to Barbara's room. Her bed had an additional mattress on it that was mechanically operated by air to turn her body back and forth. The nurses explained that it helped prevent skin breakdown. She also had what appeared to be two boots on her legs also operated by air. The nurses explained that the boots constricted to force blood back toward the heart, which would help prevent blood clots. I notice that Barbara's color looked good and her heart rate was down to 125 with blood pressure of 97/54 and a temperature of 99.5 degrees.

Tom and I went to opposite sides of the bed to talk to Barbara. Her eyes were open, but not focused. It was as if she was looking around wondering what had happened to her. When I spoke, she seemed to recognize my voice. When Tom spoke she seemed to move her eyes in his direction. We didn't know if it meant anything or if it was just a coincidence. We talked to her until she closed her eyes and drifted off to sleep. It seemed to be a peaceful sleep. Not one filled with restlessness and thrashing as I had noticed throughout the previous week. Around 2:00 PM the nurse came to suction her lungs. Barbara showed a great deal of discomfort every time this procedure occurred. Tom noticed that this time she also raised her right arm slightly. This was the first muscle reaction that we had observed since she went into the coma.

Around 3:00 PM Barbara seemed very restless. I talked to her and told her to try to get some rest. I even rubbed her feet, which seemed to soothe her somewhat. As she drifted off to sleep, I noted that this was the first time in many days that she actually seemed peaceful. The entire previous week was filled with coughing and spitting up, and she just didn't get any rest. I took a quick check of the monitor and noted that her heart rate was down to 128 with a blood pressure of 92/50 and a mild fever.

About forty-five minutes later a crisis occurred with Barbara's blood pressure. As the monitor showed a steady decrease the nurse asked us to leave the room. She then proceeded to increase the flow of IV fluids. She also raised the rate of flow of the dopamine, this was a drug used to help constrict the blood vessels, thus increasing blood pressure. Around 4:30 PM as Tom and I again sat in the room, one of the IV machines started beeping its alarm. I looked over and saw that it was the IV drip that contained the dopamine. When I saw that there was no immediate response from the attending nurse, I became alarmed. I looked at the vital statistics monitor and observed that Barbara's blood pressure was dropping quickly. The monitor showed a pressure of 77/30, and I left to get a nurse. Again she asked us to leave the room. In a short period of time the nurse came out. I asked her what was going on, and she explained that the IV line in Barbara's Hickman catheter had fallen out and the fluids were going on her chest. The nurse resolved the problem and left the room. I was really filled with anger at that time because of the lack of an immediate response by the nurse to the beeping alarm of the IV pump machine. Before she left the room she handed me a printout of the CAT scan. I asked her what it all meant and she responded that it was only an initial report and that I had to wait for the neurologist to read it later that afternoon. I took the report and looked it over. It read, "Soft tissue hematoma overlying the left temporal bone no definite intraluminal coup or contra coup injury is identified. No evidence of intracerebral hemorrhage or infarct is appreciated." To me this meant that Barbara had a small bruise and there was no evidence of any swelling or mass on the brain. I would find out later that day that I was correct. Before the nurse left the room she told me that she had put in a call to Dr. Williams because of the problems that she was having with the blood pressure.

Around 4:45 PM Dr. Williams arrived and examined Barbara. She told me that she was very concerned with the fluctuating blood pressure. She really didn't have any answers and only said that a spreading of the infection caused by the pneumonia could cause it. She asked me what I wanted done if Barbara's blood pressure fell so low that her heart stopped again. I told her that I wanted them to try to revive her. Dr. Williams was concerned that we were giving Barbara the best treatment possible and if her heart stopped again, then we would not have made any progress by simply reviving her once again. I told her that I did not care, that I wanted them to do everything possible to give her a fighting chance at survival even if we were back to the same state as before. The alternative was simply to let her die, which I wasn't ready to do at that time. This was all playing a great deal of havoc with my emotions. Two days earlier I had watched her die and now she was clearly alive. How could the doctor think I would want anything less than every possible chance at a recovery? I kept clinging to the idea that if her bone marrow produced massive amounts of good white cells to help fight off the infection, then my dear wife could have a good chance of beating the odds.

At 5:30 PM my sons decided to leave and go prepare us a meal. I told them that I was going to stay at the hospital because I was very concerned about the problems with the blood pressure. No sooner had they left than the IV pump containing the dopamine started its loud beeping alarm once again. When I looked up at the vital statistics monitor I saw that Barbara's blood pressure was falling rapidly. I looked back at the IV pump and quickly found the problem. The nurse had let the bag containing the dopamine run dry. She came into the room and I pointed out the problem to her right away. She changed the fluids and immediately Barbara's blood pressure started to rise again. I was furious with the situation but I did not say anything to the nurse. I went out of the room to the IV receptionist's desk and asked to see the senior physician on duty. In a few moments I was introduced to a Dr. Webb. I told him that I wanted to speak to him in private. We went into Barbara's room and I closed the door. I told him that I was going to try to talk to him in a logical and rational state, considering the fact that my emotions were shot at that point. I told him about my concern for the lack of immediate attention by the nurse. I went on to point out that it appeared to me that at that point the dopamine was vital to keeping Barbara's blood pressure under control and keeping her alive. He agreed with my assessment. I went on to add that if that was the case, then the nurse should pay a lot more attention to the alarms on the IV pump. I told him that I was not staying there in the room to maintain a vigil over a dying loved one; I was there because I did not trust the nurse who had failed to respond without my insistence. He assured me that he would take care of the problem. We went on to discuss the problem with so much swelling in Barbara's upper extremities. He felt that there was some kind of a blockage preventing the fluids to flow back down the body and be processed out. At the conclusion of our discussion I felt a little better. The thought kept coming to me, "What if I had left? Would I have gotten a call at home that informed me that my wife's blood pressure had fallen and her heart stopped and they were unable to revive her?" I really had some doubts about the care and treatment at that point. That is why I maintained absolute control over every decision to be made concerning the treatment of my spouse.

I left the hospital soon and drove back to Carlisle. When I got home the boys had a wonderful meal prepared. We gave a blessing to the Lord, and made our traditional toast to a higher white blood count. After dinner, we drank a few beers and talked. I knew that I was both physically and emotionally destroyed, so I went to bed early.

I got up early the next morning and called the hospital to check on Barbara's condition. The nurse told me that her blood pressure remained between 98/64 to 104/64 most of the night. Her heart rate at that time fluctuated between 120 and 130, and she had a mild fever. But the good news was the increase in the white blood cell count to 1,360. She went on to add that she was able to decrease the rate of flow of the dopamine and saline solutions, but there was some bleeding coming from the suction tube in the stomach. The nurse put in a call to Dr. Williams to inform her about the bleeding.

After getting the morning report, I drank some coffee and ate two pieces of toast. I took the dogs for their morning walk and just waited until my sons and two brothers got out of bed. Around 9:45 AM Dr. Williams called me. She said that she was not overly concerned about the bleeding in Barbara's stomach. It was common for patients in the ICU to have some mild bleeding. She explained that the suction tube could be rubbing up against the stomach lining and causing some mild irritation. Dr. Williams's major concern was the amount of upper extremity swelling and the fact that Barbara had now gone several days without any nutrition. She told me that there could be three things causing the swelling; a blood clot, the fungus infection was spreading, or a tumor from the previous cancer. Her recommended course of action was to inject some dye directly into Barbara's Hickman and track it to see if there was any blockage. The doctor also told me that Barbara's kidneys were working, but not very well. She wanted to give her some Lasix, a diuretic, to try to stimulate the kidneys. She explained that the kidneys were vital to processing excess fluids out of the body, and their weak function could be related to the fluid retention. Dr. Williams also said that they wanted to remove the catheter from the chest and put a new multiport in the groin area. This was needed to ensure that the fluids required did in fact get into the system. She told me that they would be working for several hours and that she would call me if she felt it appropriate. I told her about the problems that I had with the nurse the day before and she told me that she would look into it. I hung up the phone and decided to stay at home until at least 11:30 before departing for the hospital.

I did not receive any additional calls from the doctor, so son Tom and I left. We got to the ICU room around 12:15. Barbara's heart rate was now down to 109 with a blood pressure of 112/63. She was still running a slight fever, but I knew that it was due to the infection. The attending nurse entered the room and told us that she had to treat Barbara for a vaginal yeast infection, so Tom and I went down to the snack bar for a small lunch. When we returned to the room, we took our now usual positions beside our loved one's bed, Tom on the right and me on the left. As we spoke to Barbara we could see her rolling her eyes under the lids. It appeared that she was trying to move them toward our voices. All we said was that we loved her very much and we told her about the events of the day. We tried to talk to her in a positive voice all the time, with hope for a future. As we talked we could see Barbara struggling to open her eyes through her swollen face. She did not seem to be in any pain, but it appeared that she was in a daze and did not know what had happened to her. It was painful watching her go through all of this, but it was a condition that we had to deal with every waking moment.

About an hour later, my son Jason, brothers Steve and Pat arrived. Although it was a very emotional and morbid in the ICU room with the constant sound of the ventilator going in and out, we tried as best as we could to offer support and encouragement. After all, our wife, mother, and sister-in-law was sick and fighting for her life.

As we all sat and talked in the ICU room I kept a constant watch on the life-support monitor. It just appeared to me that there was some sort of an unexplainable correlation between Barbara's decrease in heart rate and the increase in blood pressure. It didn't make any sense, because the faster your heart beats, the more it is pushing the blood out into the veins. The nurse told me that all of the vitals got better just after they inserted the new multiport into the groin area. So maybe the new port was allowing the fluids to flow more easily. At any rate, the heart rate was now 109 with blood pressure of 118/67. The nurse was also able to reduce the amount of dopamine once again. The whole idea of decreasing it gradually was to get Barbara to a state where she maintained her own blood pressure without the assistance of drugs.

My brother Pat made a comment that the urine bag appeared to be a lot fuller than the previous day. When we asked the nurse, she concurred that Barbara was now passing a lot more urine. So it appeared for the time being that the Lasix did the job intended and should help relieve some of the excess fluids and eventually bring the swelling down.

As I sat in the room writing in my journal and watching the monitor, I couldn't stop the swarm of emotions that came over me. I felt that Barbara was making some progress. She was still critically ill and near death but there were some signs of improvement. Right after this thought I found myself thinking that I should be prepared for the eventuality of death. I am sure that I was still in some state of shock filled with a lot of anxiety, despair, sorrow, pity, hope, and a variety of other emotions. The swings between each of the emotions were almost too much to handle. I just hung on to the thought of what Dr. Williams told me a few days earlier, "Poor, but not impossible."

By 3:15 that afternoon Barbara's heart rate was 108 with blood pressure of 118/65. So it appeared that she was somewhat stable. She continued to roll her eyes around and I observed that when her sons talked to her the monitor showed an increase in blood pressure. I also watched as the nurses constantly suctioned out her lungs and used a vacuum to clean out her mouth that Barbara did not like it at all. Her blood pressure would always increase and she made strange faces like the whole procedure was uncomfortable. The nurses had to talk to her when the vacuum was in her mouth because she would bite down on it and they were unable to move it around. Again it wasn't a pretty sight, but it was the one that I had to deal with at the time. The doctors had made a decision that Barbara needed to get some nourishment, so at 5:00 PM the first of a continuous bag of Nutrimix Macro (food supplement) and Liposyn (fat) were fed intravenously. I stayed at the hospital till 9:30 that night.

After our late meal, I sat and talked to my sons and brothers. The telephone rang constantly from family and friends. I only talked on occasion because I was just mentally exhausted and could not muster up enough strength to talk to everyone. It was so good having help from my sons and brothers because they took care of most of the household chores.

July 31 was not a lot different from the previous day. My morning call to the hospital revealed that Barbara's condition remained about the same. She had a small increase in the white blood cell count to 1,460 but that was really insignificant. In the hospital that day, I noticed that the swelling seemed to be a little better around her eyes, even though it was still pretty bad. The color of the suctioned fluids from both the stomach and the lungs had not changed.

Dr. Williams's concerns remained the same, the swelling of the upper extremities and the fact that Barbara remained unconscious. The doctor told me that she felt that Barbara might not be able to regain a conscious state because of swelling on the brain. I said to her that I thought that the CAT scan proved that there was no swelling. She corrected me and said that the CAT scan only showed that there was no mass on the brain but it was inconclusive about swelling. She wanted to inject a new drug called Decadron, a blood thinner, to see if it would decrease blockage in the blood vessels. She felt this would help the upper body to pass the fluids to the rest of the body and relive some of the pressure that might have been causing some of the swelling. Dr. Williams's best guess was that the fungus infection had spread outside of the lungs into the vessels in the chest and caused the fluid flow constriction.

When the doctor left, I prayed that she was right about the infection causing the swelling. If that were truly the case, then an increase in white cells combined with the antibiotics would eventually clear up the pneumonia. And with the kidneys working properly, the swelling would go down and release the pressure on the brain and allow Barbara to regain consciousness. It all seemed so simple, but the function of the human body is very complex. All of the organs are interrelated and there is almost always a cause and effect—if one is out of whack, it eventually complicates another. Add to that the facts that cancer cells are still running around and that her bone marrow is in the infancy of rebuilding. What you get from that scenario is that the chances for a survival diminish. But I was determined to not give up.

At 5:10 that evening, Barbara's mother and her two brothers, Bob and John, arrived from Cape Cod, Massachusetts. They were only going to stay a few days, but felt that they needed to be there to add some support. Barbara's father could not come. He was eighty years old and had some medical problems and just felt that the strain of seeing his daughter in such a condition would be too much to handle.

As soon as Barbara heard the voices of her family members, she opened her eyes. Her blood pressure shot up again but quickly returned to a lower level. I told everyone that this was common with her and that she was really making some good progress. We stayed at the hospital for several more hours and finally departed.

My house was now turning into a transient hotel. Food was always available, phones were answered, and generally I did not have to worry about anything. This was so good for me because it gave me the freedom with my energies to concentrate on treatment, care, and concern for Barbara.

The first of August brought in a new month, one filled with a lot of prayer and hope—hope for a miracle recovery. I prayed almost constantly for a little break in

Barbara's medical condition. I knew that she was critically ill, but I hung on to the thought that she could still make it.

My morning call to the ICU ward revealed that things were about the same as the previous night except that the white blood cell count had risen to 2,090. At least I could see some tangible evidence that her bone marrow was producing good white cells. The count was still way below normal and I knew that the white blood cells were being consumed fighting the infection, but at least it was something progressive.

At 9:15 AM I received a call from Dr. Williams. She told me that Barbara's kidney function blood test was a little worse than the previous day. She added that the platelets continued to remain low. But on the positive side, she said that the oxygen content in the lungs was good. Her major concerns for the day were unchanged—Barbara's head remained extremely swollen and she was still comatose. She said that the next step was to get a team of neurologists involved.

I got to the hospital around 11:20 AM. Dr. Webb was in the room and we talked for a short period. He explained to me that he thought it might be appropriate to go into Barbara's lungs and get a culture for analysis. I know that Barbara heard this because she opened her eyes as if to offer a different opinion. Dr. Webb told me that they had stopped all of the antibiotics except for the amphotericin B because of the toxicity problems and the effect that they were having on the kidneys. I noticed that the urine bag still showed ample amounts of drainage. When the doctor and I finished talking, Barbara once again opened her eyes and looked in the direction of my voice. I continued to talk to her. As I spoke, I moved my head to the center of the bed and she followed my voice, by turning her head toward it. It really made me feel good. I could sense that in her awful condition that she was at least capable of hearing and did offer a small sign of acknowledgment. Remembering back to her lengthy stay for the induction therapy, I thought that something was missing in the room. I quickly realized that the TV was not on nor had it been since we came into the ICU ward. In her previous room she kept it on twenty-four hours a day. I asked her if it would be a good idea to turn on the TV. To my surprise she raised her eyebrows.

At 12:47 Dr. Phillips, one of the team of neurologists requested by Dr. Williams, arrived to examine Barbara. We all left the room while he conducted his examination. He concluded about an hour later and he and I walked down the hall for a discussion of his findings. The essence of his comments were that he felt that during the arrest there had been a definite lack of blood and oxygen to the brain that caused some damage that was still keeping her in a coma. He felt that it had been too long since the arrest and that she should not still be comatose. He said that Barbara definitely had brain activity but only for certain functions like breathing, heart activity, and pupil constriction. His plan was to get an electroencephalogram (EEG) that would measure the electrical impulses of the brain. He said that he would schedule it for the following day.

As we talked I challenged Dr. Phillips for more information and possibilities. I asked him if a person in Barbara's condition could be capable of fighting off the infection, and still remain in a coma. His response was quite different from the same question that I proposed to Dr. Williams the previous day. Dr. Williams had told me that she felt all of Barbara's problems were directly related to the infection. She felt that Barbara could not remain sick and still stay in the coma. This was not the opinion of the neurologist.

I was beginning to get a sickening feeling in my stomach. I knew that Barbara's death would be difficult to accept, but the thought of her remaining in a coma, possibly for the rest of her life, was something that I could not handle. My mind raced rapidly over the possibilities. I could see months, maybe even years of my wife lying around some hospital ward without any hope of ever regaining a conscious state, but yet being cured from the infection, and possibly even the leukemia. After a long deliberation, I decided for the time being that I would go with Dr. Williams's assessment and continue to concentrate on the most serious problem at hand, and that was the presence of the fungus infection. I just couldn't continue to live with the thought of anything worse at that point.

When I went back in the room I felt the need to try to push Barbara along a little. I leaned over her face and just kept telling her to open her eyes. "Come on," I said, "you can do it. Work on it, work real hard. I want to talk to you." She actually responded and opened them without rolling them around. I felt that this was a positive response. After I finished, Jason did the same thing with his mother. Again, she responded with open eyes. They were not focused, but at least she was responding. We all knew that she was weak, but we felt so good to see her respond to us. We also tried to get her to squeeze our fingers in her hands, but this was just asking for the impossible.

That afternoon my brothers went to the airport to pick up my sister Linda, and my mother and father. Linda had traveled from Peoria, Illinois, and my parents flew in from Leavenworth. They arrived in the ICU room around 4:30 PM. We all tried to get Barbara to open her eyes once again, but could not get a response. At one point I leaned over her and pushed her eyelids back. You could see her rolling her eyes back and forth and struggling to open them on her own. It was as if she wanted to open them so bad to see who was in the room but just did not have the control or power to do so. Regardless, I felt good just having some additional family members there to help out in their own way. We all tried our best and everyone in the room would go up to Barbara and offer encouragement. We did not know whether it did any good or not, but it was all we could do. We left the hospital around 5:30 PM and went back to Carlisle. After the traditional meal and toast to a higher white count, everyone settled in to rest for the evening. We talked and talked. We hugged and offered comfort to each other. It was an awful mess that we were all caught up in, but nowhere as bad as what my poor wife was going through. I felt so desperate and so sorry for that wonderful woman.

When I got up the next morning for my routine call to the hospital, I found my mother and father already at the breakfast table. Mom had made coffee and my dad was eating some toast. I took the dogs out for their morning constitution and then made the call. The nurse told me Barbara's vitals at that moment were a heart rate of 106, blood pressure of 146/70, and temperature of 101 degrees. She added that the white count rose to 3,820 but the platelets were low and they were going to give her some later in the day. I decided to leave for the hospital to arrive before the doctor called me for our daily meeting of the minds because I knew that the EEG would be conducted early and I wanted to be there for it.

I got to the hospital around 10:00 AM and went directly to the ICU ward. Son Tom and I tried to get a response from Barbara as we had the previous day, but nothing happened. Barbara just remained still, letting the respirator assist her breathing. The attending nurse for the day, Tammy, commented that she was not getting a lot of response either, but the urine flow remained good. In fact she said, "Barbara is peeing up a storm."

Dr. Jenkins, the third member of the team of treating oncologists, had now taken over Barbara's case. He called me from his office for a short discussion. He said that Barbara's condition was unchanged and that he would wait for the results of the EEG before proceeding any further. I asked him why the platelet count remained so low all the time. He said that the bone marrow was producing platelets, but they were being consumed so quickly with the fever and infection.

I went back to the room and the nurse told me that the team was coming to conduct the EEG and that we needed to leave for about an hour or so. Tom, Aileen, John, Bob and I all went to the snack bar for some coffee. At 11:30 the Domos family had to leave to go to the airport. It was a very emotional scene as they each said their good-byes to Barbara. Her mother and two brothers offered their best, but did not know that it would not be enough and that they would never see Barbara again on this earth.

After the good-byes my mom, dad, two sons, and sister Linda went back to Barbara's room. We all took turns standing over Barbara and offering words of encouragement. Everyone tried so hard to get a response of some sort but to no avail. The whole afternoon I just kept waiting for someone from the neurologist's team to come in and tell me about the results of the EEG. I had a bad feeling about the outcome, but I kept hoping for the best. I just couldn't believe that Barbara could get over the infection, but still remain in the coma.

By 2:00 PM that afternoon, Barbara had the following vital statistics: heart rate 105, blood pressure 139/69, and temperature 100.94 degrees. As I watched her drift in and out of a deep sleep, I felt so sorry for her. It wasn't all of the tubes and needles sticking in her body so much as it was the thought of such a beautiful, young woman being in such a terrible condition. At this point, Barbara had no control over her bodily functions. She just existed, and I did not know for how long, but I began to feel her slip away. We all worked so hard in our own way to help out. You could feel the energy flowing in the room, and a lot of prayers were offered up to God.

I know that the entire scene was playing havoc on Jason, my youngest son. I could see the frustration in his face when he received no response from his mother. He left the room to go sit for a while in the waiting room. Sensing his hurt, I followed him to the waiting room to see if he was all right. He told me that he was all right and that he had just taken a Benadryl and that he just wanted to rest a little. I hugged him and left him alone.

When I came back in the room, Nurse Tammy came in to suction out Barbara's lungs. I was disturbed because unlike all the previous times, Barbara showed absolutely no response to this uncomfortable procedure. No eye movement or facial expression. It was as if she had slipped deeper in the coma and nothing could reach here. The nurse told me that she had talked to Dr. Jenkins about adjusting the Albumin in Barbara's Nutrimix food pack to help reduce the swelling in the upper extremities. Barbara continued to process a lot of urine, but the swelling just wasn't coming down fast enough and everyone felt that all of those fluids were putting unnecessary pressure on the brain, thus keeping her unconscious. The only good news that came out of the day was that it appeared that the amount of fluids being suctioned out of Barbara's lungs was a lot less than the previous days. It also did not have that dark nasty brown color that we had seen all week. I also noticed that her temperature remained around 101 degrees most of the day. Even with the cooling blanket applied, it remained above normal. I kept trying to figure out why we could not get a response from

Barbara. I felt that maybe the presence of a fever all day may have just made her tired and not feel good.

As my mind raced back and forth, I reflected on a conversation with Mary Hoppes, an old friend of ours that we served with in the Army back in 1984. Mary had a friend who hit her head in a car wreck and remained in a coma for six months. Mary told me that it took three months before there was any kind of a response from the patient. So was I being too impatient? I just didn't have any answers. I just wanted my Barb to get better or at least show us some kind of a sign that she was making some progress. The emotional roller coaster was killing me.

By 4:00 PM I still had not seen the neurologist, Dr. Phillips. It was frustrating knowing that it had been over four hours since the EEG was taken and no one came in to talk to me about the results. I also noticed on the monitor that Barbara's fever was starting to rise again. At 5:00 PM it was up to 101.8 degrees, the highest it had been since admittance to ICU. I did not like to see this because I knew that it took away from her strength and would make her feel awful. It also plagued my mind that the infection was spreading and that she was not getting any better. Trying to keep a positive thought in my head, I decided that it could have been related to the Tylenol. Contrary to my trying to feel positive, the fever just kept rising until it got to 102.2 degrees.

At 5:45 Dr. Phillips finally arrived. He did a physical check of Barbara as I anxiously awaited his analysis of the EEG conducted earlier that day. As we started to talk he suggested that we leave the room. He just said that he felt better not talking in front of the patient. As we left Barbara's room he began his analysis by saying that the EEG did not look good. He felt that it showed less brain function than a person who is asleep. It was his opinion, based on the physical exam and the EEG, if Barbara survived the fight with the infection that she would be "neurologically impaired." When I probed for other possibilities, he acknowledged that the problem could be related to the infection and the fact that it may have spread into the spinal cord, keeping her in the coma. Dr. Phillips felt that it was too risky to do a spinal tap at this point to check for infection. So, the only way that we would ever know if he was right or wrong was for Barbara to come out of the coma.

I know that I really didn't want to hear bad news, and that is why I kept pressing for other explanations. It was something that was imbedded in my nature to seek out all possibilities, especially one that could produce positive results.

As Dr. Phillips and I concluded our discussion, I told him how Barbara responded to me the day before. He was very surprised at this. He asked me to go back in the room to see if I could get her to do it again, because it would dramatically change the diagnosis. Of course, when we went back to Barbara's room, I couldn't get her to respond to anything. She just kept her eyes closed and remained in a deep coma. I am sure that the doctor believed me, but I really felt frustrated when I tried to show him what had happened, and got no response at all. Dr. Phillips left the room and told me that he would stay in contact with the attending physician.

As I sat in the room after the neurologist left, I had an overwhelming fear come over me that Barbara would die that night. I know that it was built up as a result of seeing the fever rise, and getting absolutely no response all day. I couldn't concentrate at all. I was tired and filled with different emotions. In my journal I wrote, "It is killing me watching her lie there in the bed and go through all of this. I've noticed that as the temperature is going up, her blood pressure is going down. This whole thing has turned into a nightmare. I think that both of her sons are really pushing for her to survive, but know that she is still very sick and could die anytime. From my perspective, I've always had hope and I told Barbara that I would fight for her all the way. But I would much rather have her dead than living in a coma."

I left the hospital that night wondering whether or not I would get a call later that brought bad news. The drive back to Carlisle was lonely. I cried tears of sadness. I couldn't keep the picture of the beautiful young woman that had raised my sons out of my mind. I felt so sorry for her and so angry that she had to go through all of this. It was not a good night.

The next morning August 3, 1994, I made my usual call to the ICU ward to get the vital statistics from the on-duty nurse. The heart rate was 95 with blood pressure of 130/64. The white blood cell count was 4500 and the temperature was down to 99.5 degrees. The nurse added that the urine flow was excellent and that when she turned Barbara over to wash her back that she opened her eyes.

Tom and I arrived at the hospital at 10:38 AM. We both tried for a long time to get a response from Barbara, but did not have any luck. It was a frustrating experience since we both knew that only two days before we were able to get her to respond. The feelings of depression and frustration were only compounded by thoughts of what the neurologist had said about the possibility of massive brain damage and that she might never come out of the coma. I somehow felt that if I could get her to respond again, then her chances for recovery would be greatly elevated. I was confused. I wanted her to prove the doctors wrong and come out of the coma. We would deal with the rest of the medical problems one at a time. I had hope. I had a feeling of control if only we could get her to respond. I wanted to show all of the doctors that Barbara Brown was a tough lady who could beat all of the odds.

I kept relying on previous conversations that I had with the nurses and friends who had been through this kind of experience in the past. They all told me that it would take a lot of patience and time for Barbara to come around. My friend Ellen O'Connor, an ICU nurse in Phoenix, Arizona, gave me a lot of comfort. She pointed out that Barbara had gone through an awful lot in the past year or so. She had received massive amounts of chemotherapy, suffered through many infections and fevers, and she was now lacking nutrition. All of this had combined to upset the chemical balance in her body. It would take some time for things to get back to a somewhat normal state.

I found myself back on the emotional roller coaster once again. I used all of my strength to remain positive. Try as hard as I did though, the constant thought of one of her vital organs finally giving out plagued my thoughts. As I thought of her possible death, I reflected back on the many conversations that we had concerning her state in life. Barbara always told me that she was so grateful for having lived such a wonderful life. She thanked God every day for me, her sons, and the many blessings that she had received. I only marveled at the strength of this woman. As I watched her go through the ordeal of fighting cancer, I felt so desperately sorry for her. She was one person who definitely did not deserve the indignities that she had suffered. I reflected back over all of the complications. Three catheters had become infected, her arms were constantly bruised and swollen, she gained a tremendous amount of weight, lost her hair twice, suffered through countless needle sticks all over her body, lost a breast, and remained drained of energy most of the time. It was odd, however, that of all of these horrible things, the one that she hated the most was losing her hair. To me the loss of the hair was uncomfortable and changed her appearance a great deal, but I knew that the real beauty of that woman was inside her. I kept thinking as I watched her lie there, how much I would miss her if she died. These thoughts were mixed with the horror of having her remain alive but comatose.

Around noon I tried for ten to fifteen minutes to get a response from Barbara. I even took her shoes off and rubbed her feet, but nothing happened. All my efforts seemed in vain. I kept hearing the words of Dr. Phillips, the neurologist. I could not accept the fact that Barbara probably had some severe brain damage. I prayed that it was just the infection spreading to the spinal cord that was the cause of her remaining in such a deep coma. I remained mentally and physically exhausted. I constantly reminded myself that it was going to take time, love and a lot of patience to get Barbara healthy again.

At 2:00 PM my mother, father, son Tom, and sister Linda all arrived in the ICU room. The scene was one of everyone talking, rubbing and encouraging Barbara along. We all tried so very hard. No one was giving up hope. We each made comments about signs we saw and drew our own conclusions. It was a desperate situation. We all felt so helpless, but did not know what else to do.

I noticed that the fluid being pumped from Barbara's stomach was redder than before. This indicated increased bleeding. The nurse also informed us that Barbara had passed a stool that morning that also had blood in it. I just thought that this was the beginning of the end. I had no idea what effect the massive amounts of chemotherapy had done to her internal organs. I also knew that with a lack of exercise, nutrition, and the fact that she had been in the hospital for over six weeks, meant that physically she was a total mess. On top of all of this, Barbara's temperature continued to rise. It just seemed that all the hospital staff was doing was keeping her alive until she eventually died. I hated the idea. I hated the notion of "modern medicine" and how inadequate it really was.

By 4:15, Barbara's temperature was starting to come back down with the aid of the cooling blanket. She seemed to be somewhat stable. She was still unresponsive, and appeared to be resting in a deep sleep. Her urine flow remained good. At least I knew that one part of her body was working pretty well.

Thursday morning, August 4, I made my usual call to the hospital ward around 8:00. Barbara's white count had risen to 7,030. Her other vitals seemed good also.

Tom and I arrived in Barbara's room around 11:00 AM. To our amazement she was lying there with both eyes wide open. The swelling around her face and hands even seemed to have decreased a lot from the day before. Tom and I immediately went to her side and began giving her words of encouragement. It was such a change from the previous day. I felt a surge of hope. As I talked to her I noticed something different, she seemed to have control over her blinking. I worked out a recognition signal with her that she seemed to understand. It was simply blink once for yes and twice for no. I asked her a whole series of question and did get a response. From our rudimentary mode of communications I learned or, at least felt that I knew, that she was not in any pain and that she knew where she was. Of course it was quite evident that, even though her eyes were open, she was still in a coma. But it was a good sign, seeing that she had some motor control and was trying to respond to us.

I watched for any new movement or reaction. When the nurses suctioned out her lungs, she really frowned and moved her head in discomfort. She was also biting down on the suction tube so that the nurses had a hard time getting it down into her lungs. I felt encouraged by all of these signs. I could feel Barbara fighting. She showed more strength today. She looked as though she was starting to come around and kick up a fight. I reflected back over my drive to the hospital earlier that day. All the way there I kept asking God for a little sign to help me along. It appeared that my prayers had been answered.

By 2:00 PM that afternoon, Dr. Jenkins, the attending oncologist, arrived to examine Barbara. Dr. Jenkins spoke with a heavy accent. I found him extremely difficult to understand. He told me that his concerns were over the temperature fluctuating, the state of the pneumonia and the bleeding from the stomach. He felt that he should just keep Barbara under close observation and "maintain the course." I told him about my concerns over Barbara's neurological state and about my discussions with Dr. Phillips. Dr. Jenkins agreed that it was possible for the infection to be spreading into the spinal cord, thus keeping Barbara in a coma.

As the afternoon went on, we did not see much change in Barbara's condition. I kept a close watch on the monitor that displayed her vitals. I also watched her reactions as the nurses came in about every hour or so to suction out her lungs. Barbara was really fighting with the nurses today. Each time they suctioned the lungs she frowned and moved her head in discomfort. For the first time I also noticed that she was moving her legs in protest.

Dr. Phillips came in the room late that afternoon after 4:00 PM. I told him about Barbara's reactions throughout the day. He looked at me like he wanted to believe what I was saying but in his attempt to get Barbara to react, he received no response. The only thing that he commented on was that Barbara did blink when he moved his hand real fast toward her eyes. I knew that the doctor and I were at odds with our analysis. Maybe I was just too close to see the truth and that I was clinging to every little movement as a sign of hope. The doctor could only go on his training, similar cases and what he saw when he examined his patient. I only prayed that I was the one who was right.

When I called the hospital the next morning I got Nurse Tammy on the phone. She said, "Mr. Brown I think you are going to be very happy with Barbara's condition today." At this a huge swell of joy filled my heart. Tammy went on to tell me that Barbara was stable, with an increase in her white cell count to 7,640. She commented that Barbara had movement in all of her extremities and responded to touch. Her liver function looked better and she continued to have good urine output. The nurse went on to add that Barbara had her eyes open and was looking around the room.

I passed on the comments of the nurse to everyone at the breakfast table and could see some momentary relief in their eyes. In my heart I felt that this was the beginning. We were finally hearing some good news on the ninth day of Barbara being in a coma. Tom and I showered and quickly left for the hospital.

At 10:45 AM Barbara's heart rate was 150/66 and her temperature was 99.8 degrees. Nurse Tammy came in the room and gave me an update. She said that all of the doctors had been in and examined Barbara and were very encouraged at her progress over the past twenty-four hours. The fluid coming out of her stomach looked almost normal. The fluid from the lungs was less than the previous day and pink in color. Tom and I commented that we saw Barb doing some things that we had not observed in the past. She was now moving her head in response to the discomfort of the breathing tube in her throat. She also seemed to move her eyes more toward our voices, but slowly. I remember thinking, "She is making signs of recovery." I knew that as each day passed she would get stronger. Both Tom and I talked to her to reassure her that she was getting the very best treatment and that she was making progress. We questioned Nurse Tammy about the lack of responsiveness. She told us that the doctors had really moved Barb around a lot that morning. She felt that her patient was just tired and needed the rest. We also noticed for the first time that Barb was moving her mouth a lot today. She was opening it and moving her tongue around like she was trying to get rid of the breathing tube.

I noted at 11:50 that her heart rate was 82 with the blood pressure of 144/65. Her temp had actually gone down to 98.94 degrees. She was resting now peacefully. I was elated to see the fever decline without the use of Tylenol. As I watched her sleeping, I noticed that her color looked good. Healthy skin color was something that you always heard older people comment on as you grew up. I guess it was a sign of healing. I could only hope. I did feel, however, that for the first time my wife was going to live. All of the signs of improvement were there. I felt that the neurologist was wrong and that I would finally win the disagreement. I knew that she was still very sick, but she was on the mend. Time would tell to what extent her recovery would be, but I felt reasonably assured that at least she would get that chance.

By 2:00 PM her fever had started to rise. It was now at 100.4 degrees. Barb was also doing a lot of thrashing around. Nurse Tammy came in to the room to give her some Ativan, a sedative to help calm her down. Tammy's main fear was that her patient might damage her lungs by moving around so much with the breathing tube. Tammy took some time to explain previous cases where she watched patients come out of a coma. This was heartening to all of the family members present. Tammy said that often coma patients would fight the breathing tube and choke on it in fear as they regain consciousness. She said that it was always helpful to have friendly voices in the room when the patient started to wake to help them overcome the fear. As she explained all of this I found myself examining my emotional state. I was now convinced that Barbara would live and that she would come out of the coma. The big question was what was her quality of life going to be like?

Throughout the rest of the day, Barb remained restless. She moved her arm and legs about quite a bit. I found myself torn in emotion. I wanted to stay by her side twenty-four hours a day, just in case she came to and needed to have me comfort her. I knew however that I was not in any physical state to do that. My mind kept saying, "Gut it out, it is the least that you can do." But logic prevailed and I knew that if she came to while I was away, that I could be at her side within thirty minutes.

As I watched my family members keep vigil over our loved one, I remember thinking how valuable a solid family is to those in need of help. I could not imagine how hard it would be for people suffering without a solid support group. On Monday of the next week, Barbara's sister, Sue, was due to arrive from Phoenix to add to our support group. My son Jason had to leave on Sunday and my sister Linda would go back to Peoria on Monday. My sister Lisa and sister-in-law Sylvia were working on tickets to come to Harrisburg on next Friday, August 12. So the transient quarters on Forbes Street in Carlisle Barracks would remain functional for some time. As I sat and watched Barb that day, I thought about a conversation that I had with our next-door neighbor a few days ago. Barbara George told me that Barbara Brown was a tough lady. She said, "Barb Brown will walk out of that hospital."

August 6 started just as the same as the previous day. I called the hospital at 8:00 AM for the morning update. The nurses' station attendant gave me vitals: heart rate 90, blood pressure 140/70, and temperature 100.4 degrees. I decided to go to the shopping mall before I went to the hospital. I returned home around 9:00. My mom told me that Dr. Jenkins had called and said that they were giving Barb another two units of blood. She added that the doctor would call me back.

As I sat at my kitchen table waiting for the return call, I noticed that today was the first day that we had sunshine in some time. The temperature outside was 60 degrees. Maybe this was a sign that a change in my wife's condition would follow the weather pattern and show a ray of light toward improvement.

So I sat in the light of a new day waiting for the busy doctor to call me back. I wanted to ask him why Barbara was continuing to receive Neupogen, the drug that stimulated the growth of white cells in the bone marrow. From my notes, I recalled that during her treatment in Kansas she could only receive Neupogen for ten days. It had now been past ten days, and they were still administering it. I found my mind wondering. I went over several conversations with the doctors. Question to Dr. Jenkins: "Is it likely that Barbara will survive?" Answer: "Not likely, her condition is poor and there are lots of complications." Question to Dr. Phillips: "Is it possible that Barb could heal physically and still remain in a coma?" Answer: "Very possible." All of this haunted my every thought. Am I trying to play doctor or just look out for my wife's care? I decided that since I took charge in the beginning that this was no time to stop.

I found myself in a confused state. I was just caught up in a helpless situation where I couldn't influence the outcome no matter how hard I tried. The phone rang around 10:00 and brought me out of deep thought and self-pity.

When I asked Dr. Jenkins why Barb was still getting Neupogen, he responded that she should not and that he would take care of it. It took everything in my Christian strength to keep from saying, "You dumb ass, you are the attending physician? You should have caught this mistake instead of me." But I held back and waited for his prognosis for the day. He told me that he would maintain the current course of action for another week. He felt concerned about Barb's neurological state. He added that if there were no improvements within the next week, then we should start discussing which of the life support systems to take away. The fear immediately jumped into my heart that I might be asked to make a decision on how Barb was going to be allowed to die. I had big choices ahead. If I picked the respirator, then she would suffocate. If I chose the feeding tube, then she could starve to death. Why did I get the feeling that the doctors had given up hope? I resolved once again to fight to the end. I would not give up no matter how rough it got.

I arrived at the hospital around 11:00 AM. Barbara's condition was unchanged. At her bedside, I noticed that her arms seemed cold. I began to massage them and talked to her trying to get a response. I made a note in my journal that the stomach fluid seemed to have more blood in it that day. I found my mind racing about to future events. I thought that if she died that I would have an autopsy conducted. I wanted to know that everything had been done to help her recover. If anything was missed I wanted to know so that the corrections could be made by the hospital staff to prevent future errors. My thoughts returned to the present. I looked at her lying there with all the tubes and needles. I felt pity and helplessness. I knew that I was beginning to lose patience with all of this. I turned to the Lord in silent prayer and asked for some strength and a little sign. Fear was taking control of all of my emotions. Logic was beginning to take a backseat. I felt that the whole key to all of this now was to get Barbara out of the coma. Once again I began to work on her trying to get a response. With each passing attempt, I only became more frustrated as nothing happened. I tried to remain calm and tell myself not to give up, but it seemed pointless. Was I losing faith? Was I, too, a victim of despair and, like the doctors, knew that it was just a matter of time? I told myself to focus and get a grip of my emotions. So I turned to the physical aspect of the room and went back to writing in my journal.

I began to think about the increase of the blood in the in the stomach fluid. What did this mean? I knew that with blood loss that the pressure would begin to drop again. I also knew that the doctors could replace lost blood. But what if the stomach bleeding got worse? How would they keep up with it? I really had hoped that today, with the fever somewhat under control, that Barbara would be more responsive. But it just was not going to happen. In fact, she was so listless that I felt that she was much worse than the previous day. In the midst of all this sadness, however, I must admit that her color looked good. The old folks again!

Around 3:20 PM her temperature rose to 101 degrees. For some strange reason it always seemed to rise in the afternoon. I started to reflect over the past twenty-five years. I knew and could almost hear Barb's voice tell me that I was doing everything right for her and not to change a thing. She always did trust me, and now would be no different even though she couldn't express it. I guess it is something that two people develop over many years together that lets the other know what they are feeling with nonverbal communication. Flashbacks of a beautiful young woman kept my mind occupied. And just as I was about to go into a "pity me" mode again, the respiratory therapist came in the room to suction out her lungs.

I noted that the suctioning process was less frequent. It also appeared that the fluid was a lot clearer than yesterday. Was this the answer to my prayers for a sign? Was this the beginning of the clearing of the fungus that ravaged her body and put her in this state, or was it just wishful thinking?

Throughout the rest of the day, Barbara continued to thrash about a lot. My sister Linda and I stayed at her side and constantly assured her that it was all right. The nurse gave her some more Ativan to help her rest. After an emotional good-bye from Jason, we left the hospital around 6:30 PM.

August 7 marked the eleventh day of the coma. I made my usual call to the nurses' station for the vitals around 8:00 AM. The heart rate was 90 with a blood pressure of 112/50 and a temperature of 100.4 degrees. The nurse added that Barbara had trouble throughout the night breathing. They increased the pressure on the ventilator. I hung up the phone and turned my thoughts toward my youngest son. He had to go back to Kansas to school before seeing his mother out of danger.

We left for the airport around 9:50 AM. It was a drive through the Pennsylvania countryside that takes about forty minutes from Carlisle. The car was pretty much silent all the way to the airport. I knew where my son's thoughts lingered. I knew that he hated to go back without seeing his mother recover. Things do not always seem fair and especially when you are twenty-one years old. I tried to console him by telling him that there was nothing at the hospital that he could do other than provide moral support. He knew this, and it did seem to help. After we checked in his luggage, we talked about his feelings. His attitude toward his mother never changed. He was the youngest of the family and always found strength in his mom. He told me that he felt good about her pulling through the coma. He said that she was always a fighter, and he couldn't see her changing now. We hugged, cried, and said farewell at the ramp to his plane. I told him I would keep him informed, and to not give up hope. He returned the goodwill and departed for the plane.

14

DECLINE

The trip to the hospital from the airport took me about twenty minutes. All the way there I went over events in my mind. I prayed for strength and courage to face whatever waited in ICU room 002. I prayed for a miracle, or just a little relief and some sign of improvement for my wife. My thoughts went back to my early morning phone call to the nurses' station. "Problems breathing, we had to increase the pressure on the ventilator," kept repeating in my head. Why couldn't we get a break? Just a few days ago I saw positive signs of recovery. Now I was not so sure. I was hurt, confused, and emotionally wrecked.

I entered the hospital elevator and took several deep breaths. I never knew what I would find as I took the short walk from the elevator down the increasingly long corridor to the ICU ward. If I turned the corner and saw no bed in room 002, then I knew that the dreaded event of death had finally come. But those thoughts were quickly dampened as I saw the familiar, swollen body full of hoses. It was sad to see a once healthy and bubbly lady in such a condition.

As I entered the room and gave my routine greeting of love and concern, I saw that Barb had her eyes open and staring at the ceiling. This was the first time that she had them open in several days. I also noticed that she seemed agitated at the attending nurse who was trying to vacuum out her lungs. The nurse decided to give her some more Ativan to help her rest more peacefully. I held her hand, offered my love and support and she drifted off to sleep.

I looked over the chart and checked out the instruments in the room. Everything looked good at this point. The fever was down and both heart rate and blood pressure were adequate. The attending physician came into the room and told me that he felt that Barbara's lungs sounded wet. He ordered a series of X-rays to see if the lungs were getting worse. He speculated that an increase in the fungus in the lungs could be the reason Barbara was having difficulty breathing.

I sat in the chair beside the bed while the technicians wheeled in a portable X-ray machine and took their photographs. Around 10:50 AM, I noticed that Barbara's blood pressure was starting to drop. The doctor and attending nurse told me that this had been going on since last night and that they had to put Barb back on dopamine to control the pressure. At 10:57 her blood pressure was 70/41. I was very nervous. I kept thinking back to the time I saw her expire in room 602. I did not want to go through that again. The doctor also had the nurse increase the flow of dextrose and they added a bag of platelets. As all of this went on, I kept watching the instruments. The fever was returning. I tried to make some sense out of all of this. I asked the nurse what she thought was going on. She explained that when a patient passes a lot of fluids out of the body, then the blood pressure could fall. In Barbara's condition, it did not take much to push her off the delicate balance of life.

Sitting there by the bed, I was torn between trying to maintain a positive attitude, and not wanting to see Barb suffer any more. If God was unwilling to perform a miracle, then I was prepared for him to take her right away. I wanted both of us to have some peace, but I did not want her dead to get this peace. I wanted her to recover, open her eyes, and shout out. I did not want the memories of a lifetime to be blurred by the passing of my partner hooked up to a sucking ventilator. But I thought, if it does occur, there would be no more humiliation, no more cancer, no more chemo, and no loss of dignity. After eleven days of ups and downs my thoughts were almost constantly negative. Was I trying to fight off the inevitable?

At 11:50 Dr. Jenkins, my son Tommy, my mom, my dad, and my sister Linda arrived. I told them about the change in Barbara's condition. No one went up to her bed right away like they had in the past few days. There was silence in the room. Fear stood out on their faces. I could tell that they expected the worse to come. Eventually, they all loosened up a little and put their private thoughts aside. They all started the ritual of bedside support. I went outside to talk to Dr. Jenkins. He did not seem concerned about the change in the blood pressure. He felt that the staff could control that with drugs. His main concern was the infection in the lungs. This was and always had been the number one problem; a problem that I would later learn was not uncommon to cancer patients.

By 2:45 that day Barbara's fever had risen to 102 degrees, the highest in several days. It only reinforced Dr. Jenkins's concern. The infection was still present and probably not getting any better. Barbara's body was trying to fight off an infection with minimal white blood cells, complemented with antibiotics. It was a hard thing to do for one in a weakened state.

The nurses came in the room and removed the high-top sneakers that I had brought to the hospital to help support Barbara's feet. They placed two Styrofoam blocks on each side of the ankles and taped them in place. Little did they know that with all of the other problems, Barbara was double-jointed in both her wrists and feet. I said nothing and let them work. I asked the nurses why they were placing Styrofoam blocks on her feet. One of the nurses said that the blocks were there to support Barbara's feet, and keep them from sagging. This decreased the chances of a blood clot forming in Barb's legs.

By mid-afternoon a combination of cooling blankets, drugs and a little luck brought the fever down to 100 degrees. The respiratory therapist came in to suction her lungs. I was shocked to see a response from Barbara. She frowned in displeasure. In my heart I could hear her, telling them to leave her alone.

The rest of that day was uneventful until early evening. I noticed that Barb was really pressing down on the hospital bed. It looked like a person lying on their back who was having a tooth pulled without Novocain. Tommy and I continued our watch until around 6 PM. When Tommy was assured that his mother was resting soundly, he motioned for me to take us all back to Carlisle.

Monday morning, August 8, 1994, in Carlisle started out slow. The weather remained hot and muggy. My attitude toward events in my life was questionable. I made the normal call to the nurses' station at the hospital. The call proved to be routine. No change in Barbara's condition. I showered and got ready for the drive to the hospital.

Tommy and I arrived at the hospital around 10:30 AM. I noticed that Barb's color looked good. Upon hearing our greetings, she seemed restless and began thrashing around in the bed. She pushed down on the bed with her hands and moved her head from side to side. To me, it seemed that she was trying hard to come out of the coma, but just did not have the strength to make it.

Nurse Kathy came in the room and told me the plans for the day. I told her that I would like to see the ICU attending physician. My main concern remained the infection in the lungs. I wanted another opinion. I found myself constantly looking for any signs of hope. I felt that an outside doctor unfamiliar with the case might have a different opinion that might prove successful. Nurse Kathy continued to say that Dr. Jenkins had ordered two more units of blood. I felt reassured that the staff was doing all they could to make a very sick patient well once again.

As I sat at the bedside, I found my thoughts once again wandering. I felt that things were improving, even though there were no tangible signs. My role for that day was to buck up strength and continue support. I had confidence in Barbara's ability to overcome the toughest odds. It was my role to see to it that she did. I knew that it was going to be a long battle after she came out of the coma. It would take a lot of time, patience, and love to make it work. I just knew that things were going to get better. What I did not have was a strong visible sign. Where was the needed break that I prayed for constantly? I felt that the worst was over. After all, there were no signs of a failing heart, kidney, or any other major organ. This seemed to me to be a good sign after twelve days in a coma. I knew, however, that the infection in the lungs had to be dealt with and cleared. This remained the primary point of focus.

Soon Dr. Hattok, the ICU attending physician, arrived. My discussion with him was not revealing. He felt that the infection in the lungs had to be eliminated if there were to be any hopes of a full recovery. He said that the staff had to increase the pressure on the ventilator to help Barb breathe easier. Everything else remained the same. When I asked about changing the antibiotic to fight the infection, he responded that it was not an option at this time. He did not want to upset an already delicate balance of chemicals rushing around Barbara's body. I finished my conversation with Dr. Hattok and returned to the ICU room. After checking the vital statistics, I decided to leave for the evening around 8:00 PM. I spent the rest of the evening having dinner with my son, parents and sister-in-law. We talked over the events of the day until exhaustion overcame me and I went to bed.

Malcolm and Molly, our two black Schnauzers, got me up early for their morning walk. While eating some toast and drinking coffee, I called the nurses' station. The morning report was not unusual, although the white blood count did drop to 5,500 from the previous day's 6,100. I remember Dr. Jenkins telling me that this was normal, due to the body trying to fight off the infection. I wondered at the time what would have happened if we had not agreed to the chemotherapy for the leukemia. What are the results of not taking a drug that destroys your immune system and makes it virtually impossible to fight off a serious infection? This was something that I did not ask the treatment team before the decision was made to go into the hospital for treatment. It would certainly be something, however, that I would investigate later. Some time after she was gone, I did look into it and learned that if she had not taken more chemo, she would have died from cancer. It was a catch-22.

I arrived at the hospital at 10:15 AM accompanied by Tommy and Sue, my sister-in-law. A new nurse named Sharon was on duty in ICU room 002. She told us that the EEG team had just finished and that the neurologist would be in later in the afternoon to read the results. We each took our place beside Barbara and noticed that she was resting peacefully. This was a different state from the previous day when all she did was seem to fight with the ventilator tube.

My attitude that day was one of hope and support. I felt that we had been through too much to give up. I tried real hard to put the past events behind me and concentrate on the present. It felt good that Barbara was resting peacefully. It seemed to me that the restful state gave her body more time to heal without using up her energy.

I was anxious to talk to the neurologist, but knew from past experience, that I would have to wait until late in the day when the team made their rounds to the hospital. I also began to think about my status. My support team was going to start to diminish. My sister-in-law was due to leave the next day and Tommy had to leave on Friday, August 12. That would leave only my parents. I felt good that everyone had had the chance to come and try to help out, but I was saddened that Barbara's eldest son, like his brother, would have leave before seeing his mother come out of the coma. I felt that my primary duty was to stay at Barbara's bedside, but I had to go back to work at some point. Her overall condition did not seem to change. She did not get any worse or better. So, I felt that I should go to work in the mornings and spend the afternoons and evenings with my mate. No one knew how long this might go on, so I decided to return to work the next Monday, August 15.

At 11:10 AM one of the attending pulmonary doctors asked to talk to me in the ICU waiting room. He told me that during the previous evening around 10:00 PM Barbara had pushed the ventilator tube out of her throat. The doctors and nurses were able to get it back down with no complications. I reflected over the previous day's restless activities and Barbara's apparent discomfort with the ventilator tube. I could not figure out how she pushed the tube out. After all, she was weak, in a coma, and the tube was taped with white adhesive all around her head and face keeping the tube in place. Somehow, her agitation got the best of the tube. Although the situation was not at all funny, I do remember a silent chuckle about the incident. It was just so typical of Barb. When she was pissed at something, she usually took action. The inside laugh that I had, brought some hope and encouragement for the day.

The rest of that afternoon was routine. We each took our turn offering words of encouragement and support. The nurses came and went doing their daily duties until their shifts changed. I monitored the instruments for any sudden changes and continued to make notes in my journal. At one point around 2:45 PM Barbara's blood pressure dropped to 74/48. The response from the nurses was to increase the flow of the dopamine. They also gave her some Tylenol to help bring down the ever-advancing fever.

At 3:25 PM Dr. Jenkins arrived for his daily check. He remained quiet and went about his work, mainly checking over the statistics posted on his patient's chart. Dr. Jenkins handed me the report from the neurologist who had examined Barb the previous day. The report summarized that her mental condition was being tied to her physical state. If her physical state did not improve, then the doctor surmised that the neurological condition had no chance of improving. He ended his summary of my wife's condition by stating that her condition was "poor," but due to her age, it was not impossible for her to recover. I handed the report back to Dr. Jenkins, and once again had an internal smile to myself. I thought back to a conversation that I had with Dr. Williams two weeks before where she described Barb's condition as "poor, but not impossible." I recalled telling her that the phrase was a double negative and I would rather hear, "poor, but possible." Did these two doctors have the same instructor in medical school who taught them how to deal with a patient's loved ones? It appeared to me at the time that doctors fit in the same category as lawyers. When it came to talking to "lay" people, they would rather use jargon than common English. Thus, the internal smile.

Throughout the rest of that afternoon, Barb remained unresponsive to our pleas for some recognition of any kind. As we all tried to comfort her in our own way I placed a pillow under her swollen arm to take off some of the pressure of the weight. When I lifted her arm to put the pillow under it, I noticed that she seemed disturbed and that she looked up to see who was moving her about. I did not like the fact that I had apparently disturbed her peacefulness, but I did enjoy seeing her open her eyes and respond to an external stimulus.

We remained at the hospital that day until 6:00 PM when we left for Carlisle Barracks. We had our nightly prayer, glass of wine toast to a rise in the white blood cell count, and then just relaxed until bed. I could tell, from the silence in the little Army quarters, that the emotional strain was playing havoc with everyone.

Wednesday morning, August 10, 1994, started out just like all the previous days since my wife had gone into a coma. I made the call to the nurses' station to get the vitals, and see how the patient did the previous night. Before I left for the hospital, I received a call from my best friend, Jack O'Connor, who lived in Phoenix, Arizona. The checkups as he called them, had now become part of my daily ritual. He asked about my physical state, and voiced a concern that I would be no good to Barbara if I got too sick to help her. I told him that I appreciated his concern, but reinforced that it was just something that I would have to work through. I was committed to keeping a vigil and nothing would stop me.

Tom and I arrived at the hospital at 10:00. Somehow with him by my side in the elevator I did not feel the need to make that prayer that I would find someone alive in ICU room 002. We made our trek down the corridor and into the room. I noted in my daily journal that swelling to the upper extremities had returned. When I asked the nurses for an explanation, they felt that the increase in fluids via the IVs to help control the fluctuations in the blood pressure was probably the answer. The lung secretions remained the same; yellow with traces of blood. The stomach secretions looked greenish with no signs of blood. Barbara continued to rest peacefully without any response to the respiratory therapist when she suctioned out her lungs. Barb was simply listless that day. All of this concerned me and mixed up my thoughts. On one hand I wanted some signs of struggle and movement that would indicate a possible break from the coma. On the other hand, I felt that her best chance of healing was to rest and let her body, supplemented with medication, clear up the infection. I thought back to the time I had bacterial pneumonia. I remembered that all I wanted to do was sleep. Maybe I had the answer to my anxieties for the day. So, I took a seat and reflected over the many years of our life together. I wondered what prognosis of the neurologists would play out after her recovery. Would Barbara Brown be a different person? How would she react to all of us? Would she be angry if she did not have all of her motor functions restored? What if she recovered, but did not know any of her family? What if she beat the odds to only have another form of cancer come again in a few years? These questions plagued my mind. But none of this would happen, at least not until she got rid of the pneumonia and came out of the coma. I thought about the previous day's conversation with Dr. Jenkins. He was concerned over the erratic nature of Barb's platelet count. He said that he might go back for some more marrow to see if the presence of cancer still existed in the bone. He went on to indicate that the team would look for some progress by the end of the week. If there were no visible signs of improvement then they would like to discuss "options." I cut that conversation off quickly because I knew that these options would involve my decision to take Barbara off some of the life support. I was in no mood to discuss those things at that time. I was determined to stay the course. Either my wife got better and came out of the coma or we would treat her as long as she could breathe on her own with the support of the ventilator. I was not going to allow any doctor the opportunity to play God. We would give Barbara every chance possible. I just could not bear looking at the future without my wife, who might have had a chance to live if we'd allowed nature to take its course.

Just as my anger toward the cancer and Dr. Jenkins reached a climax, he entered the room. I tried to ease my thoughts and let him do his daily examination. Afterward, he told me that he felt that Barb was jaundiced and that he would order a blood test to check her liver function. He tried to tie several events together to explain changes in Barbara's condition. He was concerned that her nose was bleeding and the fact that the platelet blood count was erratic. He explained that the liver was the organ that helped the blood to clot. To me it was just one more little irritant to worry about. I asked for the report from the neurologist who had ordered the second EEG the day before. The notes had "low and slow" jotted down in the typically poor penmanship of a medical doctor.

After Dr. Jenkins left, the pulmonary team came in to work on getting the amount of pressure on the ventilator decreased. They explained to me that the longer a patient is on a ventilator the more likely it is that lung damage would occur. They were afraid of puncturing an already weakened organ. They managed to reduce the pressure from 60 breaths per minute to 44. Tommy and I were asked to leave the room while a second team came in to conduct a sonogram of Barb's stomach. The nurses said that they wanted to check for kidney stones. I thought to myself, that there seems to be a lot of concern over the kidneys. Was this the beginning of a major organ failure? I wiped the thought away quickly and took my son for some lunch.

The rest of the afternoon was pretty uneventful. We saw the usual afternoon rise in temperature and the nursing staff's fight to maintain good blood pressure. Before we left for the day, the attending nurse told me that the results from the blood test for liver function all proved to be in the normal range. At least I had one thing to be thankful for that evening.

Tommy and I made the drive back to Carlisle Barracks with a slight deviation. I took him to a little town called Boiling Springs, the site of the Yellow Breeches River and one of Pennsylvania's most famous trout streams. We walked along the riverbanks and threw stones. It almost seemed like a normal day. The sun was warm and the water refreshing. For a brief moment, we were both able to escape.

That evening I got a call from Jenny Saltness, a friend for many years. She told me a story about a friend who had a heart attack and was out for ten to fifteen minutes before the medics were able to revive him. When they got him in ICU, he had another heart attack and became comatose. The doctors opened him up and performed a bypass operation. The patient lived through the operation but remained in a coma for five weeks. A year later he was fine and fishing in Minnesota. Jenny told me to hang in there and not give up hope. I told her that I appreciated her advice, and that I was taking everything one step at a time.

15

FINAL DAYS

Thursday, August 11, started out as a better day. The morning was muggy from the previous two days of rain, but the sun was shining brightly. As I took the dogs for their morning walk, I took in the warmth of the sun. I thanked God for everything that he had given me, and asked him for a little relief for my wife's suffering. I truly wanted this horrible nightmare to be over. I prayed for strength and perseverance. I also asked God to grant a little miracle. I did not have to give him the specifics.

At the end of the walk I made my call to the hospital. The nurse told me that the previous evening went pretty well. She said that Barbara had rested most of the night. I asked about the blood pressure and was told that it was steady, but they were still using dopamine to control it.

Tommy and I arrived at the hospital at 10:20 AM. Barbara's condition looked about the same. But her lips were swollen and cracked; the nurses now had applied gauze to them to soak up the blood. Beside that, her color looked good and she seemed peaceful.

At 11:05 AM a nurse named Grace came into the room and gave me an update. When she concluded, I asked her about the amount of Ativan that the doctors were still ordering to help Barbara rest. It just seemed to me that when Barb fought the breathing tube she got more Ativan. When she got more Ativan, her blood pressure would drop, and then the staff had to increase the amount of dopamine to bring the blood pressure back up. This was a cycle that I thought should be avoided. I was not trying to play doctor by any means, but with so many people trying to do so many things I wanted to make sure that no mistakes were being made. Nurse Grace told me that she would recommend to Dr. Hattok to decrease the amount of Ativan. I also asked the nurse to get me some information from Barbara's file concerning the morning of July 27, the day that she went into the coma. My concern centered on the type of drugs administered that day and the reaction of the blood pressure. I wanted to see if there was any correlation between recent events with the Ativan and the dopamine.

Nurse Grace returned to the room about ten minutes later with the information that I had requested. She told me that on July 27 Barbara had received cough syrup with codeine, Darvocet for pain, and some Zantac for heartburn. Her blood pressure at the time was 100/62. She went on to add that upon examination by Dr. Williams that morning, the doctor ordered an increase in the amount of fluids to help bring the blood pressure up. I took this all in my head and did a quick analysis. It appeared that all of the procedures conducted on that fateful morning were correct. I felt somewhat relieved, but still cautious. I had to continue to play the role of medical police. It was one of the things that kept me going. I always kept in mind that critical day when one of the nurses let the dopamine drip run dry. I was determined to do all I could to make absolutely sure that no mistakes were or would be made. I had known all my life that the best manager of one's destiny was one's self. In the case of my critically ill wife, she had no one to manage it but me.

By late that afternoon, the problems with blood pressure and fever returned. The mood in the room was somber. We continued to keep the shades closed on the window. We kept the lights dim and only turned them up when one of the medical staff arrived for an examination. The only noise present as Tommy and I sat by the bed was the soft hush of the ventilator pushing fresh air into Barb's lungs. My mood that day was sullen. I felt no anger. I just remained passive and numb. I tried hard to come to grips with the reality of the situation. I wanted some relief. I wanted the whole thing to go away and give us back our normal lives. I had been through so much sorrow and pain in the past two years that I was really getting sick of it all. I found it hard that day to generate any hope. I knew that at any moment I could see all the instruments go flat line. To me that was not the answer I wanted. I thought back to the day that I saw Barb die only to be brought back again. I had never been in a situation like that before. I thought, "How fragile we are." One second you are talking to someone and in the next breath, they are dead. I did not want to go through that again. I turned my attention to my son to get out of the painful thoughts of that day. I knew that he had to leave the next day and go back to work in Oklahoma. I knew that it would be a long and hard trip for him to make alone. I also thought about my own status. I had been on leave from the Army for over two weeks. I felt that I needed to go back to work because I had no idea how long Barbara would remain in the ICU. I felt that I could work a little in the mornings and spend the afternoons at the hospital.

The silence was broken at 2:25 PM when the attending nurse entered the room. She took two Tylenol and dissolved them in water. She then took the mixture and pushed it through the IV tube. This in conjunction with the cooling blanket was the procedure now used to help keep the fever under control.

Dr. Jenkins arrived at 3:30 for his daily check. When he finished we had a conversation about the check for more cancer cells in the bone marrow. I reinforced my position to him about not changing the course of treatment and he understood. Before he left, he told me that the results of the previous day's sonogram were negative. I suppose that I got a small answer to my prayers for the day. At least there were no new complications that I had to worry about. I just had to prepare myself for the departure of my son, Tommy, the next day. I was not looking forward to this good-bye.

The next morning, Friday, August 12, we got out of bed at our usual time. While I went about my daily routine with the dogs and phone calls, Tommy showered and packed his suitcase. We left the house around 9:00. Tommy wanted to stop by the hospital to say good-bye to his mother. It was a very emotional event watching him hugging his mother, tears streaming down his face and offering her words of love and support. At that point I wanted that miracle to happen more than ever. I wanted Barbara to sit up and shout out. I wanted all the pain and suffering in our family to stop. But in my heart, I knew that it was not meant to be that day.

The trip to the airport was silent as we both reflected on the sad farewell. We arrived at the departure gate, hugged, and offered each other words of support. I told my son that no matter what happened with his mother, she would always be with us. The love and family bonds that we developed over the years were something that no one could ever take away. I watched him walk down the jetway, just like his brother had only a few days before. I hated the thought of him not being there with me, but he had no choice.

By the time I got back to the ICU, Barbara's temperature had risen to 102 degrees. The nurse staff turned up the cooling blanket and administered some more Tylenol. The pulmonary staff made some changes to the ventilator. Barbara's oxygen exchange rate had dropped from the 99/98 percent range down to 89 percent. The staff explained to me that they had moved the ventilator tube and that Barbara was having some bronchial spasms, which decreased the oxygen exchange rate. When they finished their work I watched the instruments indicate an increase in the exchange rate.

I found myself very tired that day. I was now having a hard time getting a good night's sleep. I would wake often with anxiety attacks. I would lie there praying and hoping for a change in my wife's condition. As I sat in the room I kept watching Barb's blood pressure go down. The alarm on the IV drip brought the nurses to solve the problem. All they could do was increase the flow of dopamine. I could not help but wonder why the problem with the blood pressure was coming back. Barb had been stable for so long, now it all seemed to be going wrong. There were no signs of improvement. I kept repeating in my mind, "patience, love, and time." It was all I could do to keep my focus on the problem at hand.

I left the room for about thirty minutes while the pulmonary team took another X-ray of Barbara's lungs. When I returned they told me that there was no change. She still had a massive infection. This was not good news to end my day at the hospital.

Saturday morning came too early. I did not sleep well and I was upset over the bad news at the end of yesterday. My call to the nurses' station did not help matters. I was told that Barbara had too much carbon dioxide in her blood. The only good news in the conversation was that the white blood cell count was now 9800. I thought to myself, "Where was the great white cell count when we needed it most?" The answer was obvious. The white cells were killed off by the chemotherapy. It all seemed like such a barbaric way to go about business.

My phone rang at 9:40 AM. It was a call from Drs. Jenkins and Carr. The news was not good. They were concerned about the increase of carbon dioxide in Barbara's blood. They felt that the lungs were not operating properly. They had increased the ventilator pressure as high as it could go without rupturing her lungs. They also said that Barb could have leaking capillaries, which would cause more fluid to be deposited on the lungs. The recommended actions to solve this new problem were to administer a muscle relaxer that would immobilize her, and to give her some additional antibiotics in case there were other bacterial infections in the body. Dr. Jenkins finished the conversation by stating that he would order another bag of platelets to help stop the bleeding from her mouth. His final words to me were, "It is touch and go at this point."

I was devastated by this news. It appeared that the end was coming, and not the way that I had hoped it would. I kept thinking about our two sons. They would be so hurt. They believed in their mother's capacity to recover. I knew that, barring a miracle, at this point that she would never recover. I had less and less hope.

With this news I had to get away by myself for a moment. I walked down the street to the mailroom. On my way home I ran into some old friends, Jon and Jenny Moilanen. When I greeted them I broke down and cried. I hugged them both and told them that Barb was not going to make it. We all cried for a bit and then I left. I just did not know what to do at that moment. I told my parents that things were starting to go down hill rapidly and that I just could not go to the hospital right then and sit there and watch her die once more. I needed something to do. I just could not sit idle, so I decided to cut the grass.

While cutting the grass I actually think that I felt some relief. The noise of the mower and the sweat from my toil probably helped. While pushing the mower I stopped in my tracks with the strangest feeling. A feeling of complete peacefulness and joy swept over me. I could see Barbara's image in my mind, and I heard her voice call out, "I'm free sweetie, I'm free." I looked at my watch and noted that it was 11:25 AM. The peacefulness ended and I once again heard the roar of the mower. I finished my task and went inside clearly expecting to see a message on the answering marching that would reveal that Barbara had died at exactly 11:25 AM. To my disappointment, the machine had no new messages. I did not know what to think or do at that point. Was I hallucinating? Was it wishful thinking to get it all over with? Or did it really happen and the doctors just had not found their dead patient yet? One thing remained for sure for me. I now had to go to the hospital and see for myself.

When my parents and I arrived at the hospital, I was sure that I would find a dead woman in room 002. But to my surprise, Barbara was still alive. She was completely motionless. The only indicators of life were the monitors that continued to show a heart rate and blood pressure. Her appearance now was a mess. She was completely swollen up again and blood oozed from under the gauze pads on her mouth. The nurse apologized to me for her appearance, but added that she was doing her best to keep Barb clean. It was 3:00 PM, and I noticed the strangest thing. Her usual afternoon fever was not present. Her temperature was lower than the normal 98.6 degrees Fahrenheit. As I looked around the room, I noticed that the color of the secretion bowl from the lungs was bright red, indicating a lot of bleeding from the lungs. I remained calm but numb trying to put it all together in my head. I knew that the end was near and I just felt so sorry for my poor wife that she had to die looking such a mess. It was pitiful the condition that the horrible disease of cancer had brought about.

We sat in the room for an hour or so before we decided to go home. During that time I kept going over in my mind what Barbara's message meant when she told me, "I'm free." Did she mean free from life, free from cancer, free from this world or just free as in a free spirit? I still had that vision of her in my head. Her hair blowing in the breeze with that beautiful smile letting me know that everything was now going to be all right. I sat there wondering what it was going to be like living alone. Sure, I had two sons, but they had their own lives to live. I knew that the next few months were ones that I did not want to face. I motioned to my parents that it was time to go. We stopped off at the local Pizza Hut for supper. When we returned home, my first glance was toward the answering machine. The answering machine had no messages waiting. The end had still not come.

Sunday, August 14, was the last day that I would see Barbara alive. The call to the nurses' station that morning did not reveal that any miracles had taken place overnight. I waited all morning for a call from the doctors and did not receive one. Finally, at 1:30 PM, I decided to drive over to the hospital to get a firsthand account. I had sworn to myself that I would not sit in the room and wait for Barb to die. But I was filled with guilt for giving up hope and trying to stay away until the doctors called me and gave me the bad news. I really did not know what to do anymore. So I just acted on instinct.

The scene in ICU room 002 was that same as the day before. Barbara remained paralytic from the muscle relaxer. She still had a lot of bleeding coming from her mouth. Her lips were now open sores and drained all the time. She remained swollen, but her color oddly enough looked pretty good.

At 2:50 Dr. Jenkins called me at the hospital. He had been occupied with other duties and just then got around to returning my call. He told me that Barbara's potassium count was too high. He also was concerned about the fluctuations in the blood pressure. This along with a constant shortage of platelets could cause the kidneys to deteriorate. He said that he ordered the nurses to cut back on the Nutrimix pack because of the high quantity of potassium. I asked him why they just didn't order a food pack without potassium. He agreed and said that he would notify the pharmacy and start the procedure the next day. I hung up the phone and shook my head in wonderment about this doctor's abilities. I was sure he knew what he was doing, but it always seemed to me that I had to be the one to ask too many questions to solve some very simple problems. By the time I returned to the room, the nurse had already contacted the pharmacy and told me that the food pack without potassium would start at 4:30 that day.

By this time I had very little patience left and not much more hope. I knew that Barbara was starting to go down fast and that it would be just a matter of time. I remember looking at the heart monitor and thinking how strong her heart was. I knew that it would be the last thing to quit on her. She would probably have complications with the kidneys and then she could not process out all of the toxic chemicals running around in her body. I asked one of the doctors in the ICU about using the dialysis machine to help the kidneys. I was told that Barbara's problems with blood pressure made it impossible to use dialysis.

I sat in the room staring at the machines and the woman in the bed who had given me such joy for so many years. It hurt terribly to see her in such a horrible physical state, but I knew that the inner beauty and spirit of her soul was something that would last forever. I wrote in my journal some final thoughts: "The human body is so wonderful, but a very complex piece of machinery. So many functions of the body are interrelated."

I ended my final visit to the hospital's ICU room 002 around 4:00 PM. There was just nothing anyone could do to change the outcome of predicted events. I left with the reality that it was over and that Barbara Dean Brown would soon pass away. It was a heavy burden to bear. I guess that it was at this point that I knew for sure there was no more hope. It had to end in death. I said my final good-bye and left for Carlisle.

That night I had a hard time sleeping. I did not feel guilty for giving up; I was just restless waiting for the final phone call. I got up the next morning at my usual time. I made the call to the nurses' station only to find that there was no change in Barbara's condition. I decided that I needed something to get my mind off the tragedy that was about to unfold, so I got dressed in my Army uniform and went into my office. All of my coworkers were aware of the situation and they offered comfort and support. I made a few phone calls and tried to concentrate on business. Around 10:30 AM Dr. Carr called me at my office. He said that Barbara was showing signs of multiple organ failure. He told me that if a person has two organs fail that there was a 35 percent to 45 percent chance they could survive. If a person had failure in three organs, the odds became 90 percent that he or she would die. The doctor summarized Barbara's condition by stating that she had kidney, lung, and marrow failure and that she was bleeding from the stomach. It was obvious what was beginning to happen.

After I received that phone call, I decided to leave the office and go spend the day with my parents. We had some lunch and sat out on the patio talking. It was August 15, 1994, a feast day in the Catholic Church celebrating the Assumption of Jesus' mother Mary into heaven. I thought what an appropriate day for my wife to die and go to God.

I made a call to the Pennsylvania Society of Cremation in Harrisburg. They were considerate and sympathetic. About an hour or so after my call, a pleasant gentleman arrived at my quarters to explain all the procedures and have me sign the necessary paperwork.

The rest of that day was just a day of nothing. I felt hurt and betrayed. God did not grant me the miracle that I had asked for over and over again. I was not angry with God; I kept telling myself that it just was not His will to save Barbara.

I found that it was hard to accept that my closest friend and spouse was about to leave me forever. Was it an act of faith that I accepted God's will? I suppose it was. The evening rolled around without the final announcement from Dr. Smith. I needed some sleep so I went to bed.

At 12:50 AM, the phone rang. It was Dr. Smith calling from the hospital. He was brief and offered his condolences. I hung up the phone and sat on the side of the bed for a moment. I picked up the phone and called back to the hospital. I forgot to ask the doctor the time of death. The nurse told me that Barbara died at 12:35 AM, not quite on the Feast of the Assumption, but close enough.

I continued to sit on the side of the bed for several moments. I had the strangest feeling come over me again just like I had several days ago while cutting the grass. I could not see anything, but the warmth and joy surrounding my body was incredible. It seemed like I received a telepathic message from Barb telling me that it was all right and that she had to go. I believed that God had finally taken her spirit to heaven.

I heard my parents walking around so I got dressed and went downstairs to tell them the bad but expected news. My father asked me if I was all right, and I responded with a short yes. I made the calls to my two sons and asked my parents to notify the rest of the family. I excused myself, went to my bed, and cried until I fell asleep.

16

A NEW LIFE FOR ME

Early Tuesday morning, August 16, 1994, I got out of bed with a different set of circumstances in my life. I had to deal with all the preparations of burying a spouse. I did have the comfort and support of my parents who stayed with me through the whole ordeal, but I was the one who had to make the arrangements. The phone in my Army quarters did not stop ringing all day long with family and friends calling to offer their condolences. I found myself somewhat dazed and found it difficult to accept that Barbara was finally gone. Jack O'Connor called to check on me just as he did for the past month. He wanted to know if I felt relieved. I told him that I didn't feel any relief, but I did have a new focus. I now had to make all the arrangements for Barbara's memorial service back in Leavenworth. I also had to start thinking about clearing up a lot of other things such as life insurance, credit cards, driver's license, Social Security, military identification cards, health insurance, and the disposition of personal effects.

I once read an article that said not to make any decisions about anything after a spouse's death, but some things have to be acted on immediately. It is beneficial to have family and friends as part of a support group during this time. I was fortunate because I also had my military support group that included my boss, the staff at the Army War College, and my Army buddies scattered throughout the country. One of the calls that I made that day was to Colonel Mike Corbell, stationed at Fort Hood, Texas. I asked him if he would go to Leavenworth early and liaison for me with the Army staff there to set up some billeting for some relatives who would be in town to attend the memorial service scheduled for Friday, August 19. Another call went out to Father Charlie McGlinn to arrange details for the service. He told me that he would make arrangements and that he would like to meet with my two sons and me as soon as we got back to Leavenworth. I talked to Pennsylvania Society of Cremation in Harrisburg and asked if I could leave Barbara's remains in Pennsylvania until I returned from Kansas. They were most polite and stated that it would not be a problem. The gentleman that I spoke to also offered his condolences and wanted to know if there was anything else that they could do to assist me. I thanked him for his kindness and said that I would be back in Harrisburg in about two weeks to pick up the ashes.

My parents and I spent the rest of the day making our travel arrangements. We sat out on my brick patio after lunch, drank a few beers, and just talked. We went out for dinner that night and decided to turn in early to bed.

I think that day I was just numb. My emotions were just about shot. I was physically worn out from all the worry and stress, and I did a lot of praying. I talked to Barbara as if she could hear me. I felt lonely and abandoned. I had the gut-wrenching sickness that one gets when you lose a loved one. I also failed to write in my journal that day. I just felt that there was no use in continuing to write because it was all over. Much to my surprise, Barbara's fight with cancer was ended but my fight with grief was just beginning.

The next morning we all got up early to make the trip to the airport. The weather in Carlisle was cold and it was raining hard. Before I left for the airport, I got out my journal and noted that I had failed to jot any entries for the previous day. I realized that I needed that daily ritual to give me something to do to help ease the pain. So, I started the practice back up again. I wrote:

> "I am waiting for my ride to the airport. It will be a sad journey to pay my respects to Barbara, but I know family and friends will honor her. Friday is not a day that I look forward to at all. Last night I changed my mind about getting rid of the two dogs. I can still hear Barb saying, 'Don't get rid of my doggies.' I will love them and keep them. I think that they will be good company in the days ahead. My emotions now are sporadic. Sometimes I fight to clear my head and think logically. I'm very, very hurt and sad. It's as if I'm the only person on earth who ever lost a wife. I know that in time I will begin to slowly heal. I must always remember not to make emotional decisions too quickly. The next few months will be extremely hard to go on with my life. Everything in this house has Barbara's touch on it except my computer room. I find myself walking around in a daze most of the time. When I come back from Leavenworth I must get busy right away. I'll get a fence put up for the dogs and rejoin the golf club. But for now I'm just going to have to learn to suffer a little."

The trip back to Leavenworth was indeed sad, but I slept most of the way. I took up residence at my parents' house along with my two sons. I had already written out an obituary and selected a photo for the paper, so all I had to do was drop them off at the *Leavenworth Times.*

OBITUARY

Barbara D. Brown, Harrisburg, Pa., died Tuesday, August 16, 1994, in Harrisburg. She was 45.

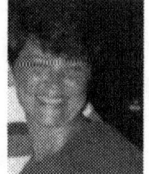

Barbara Brown

She is survived by her husband, Col. Thomas E. Brown Jr., Carlisle Barracks, Pa.; two sons Tom Brown, Miami, Okla., and Jason Brown, Lawrence; her parents, Bob and Aileen Domos, Cape Cod, Mass; two brothers, Bob Domos, Boston, and John Domos, Cape Cod, Mass.; one sister, Susan DeGeorge, Phoenix, Ariz.; her father-in law and mother-in-law, Tom and Grace Brown, Leavenworth; and eight nephews and eight nieces.

Visitation will be from 10 to 11 AM Friday at Sacred Heart Church, Leavenworth.

Memorial services will begin at 11 AM Friday, August 19, at the church with Father Charles McGlinn officiating. A reception at the parish hall will follow.

The family requests no flowers. Memorials may be given in her name to Immaculata High School.

That evening, Father Charlie McGlinn came by the house to talk with my two sons and me. We went over the details of the memorial service and picked out the readings and the music. He had managed to get a Pentecostal choir from a nearby church. That would fulfill one of Barbara's last wishes on not having morbid music at her funeral.

The next day was Thursday, the day before service. People stopped by all day long bringing food and flowers. Mike Corbell made several trips to the airport for me to pick up relatives and get them settled. The house was full of people. Most of the day we just gathered outdoors on the patio, talking. Everyone there had a story to tell about Barbara. I took some time to walk around and talk to Barbara's dad. He was distraught and needed a lot of support. As we walked, cried, and hugged each other, I could feel that I was helping him with all of his grief. He gave me counsel and said that I had to rebuild my life and move forward. He mentioned that if Barbara's mother, Evva had not died, he never would have had the wonderful relationship and marriage to his wife Aileen. I knew the message that he wanted me to take away, but it was difficult to acknowledge that he was right.

Friday came much faster than any of us wanted it to. My family and I arrived at the church around 9:30 AM and stood in the aisle outside the pews just short of the altar. From 10:00 to 11:00 we greeted all the guests that came to attend the memorial. I told my sons that a lot of the people coming up would not know what to say. I said that they should just hug them or shake their hand and thank them for coming.

The line of people waiting to greet us stretched out into the steps of the church. There were people there that I had not seen for over twenty-five years. Old friends and new ones stopped by one-by-one to say a few words. Some of them said nothing; they just hugged and cried before they went on to their seat.

At 11:00 AM Father Charlie started the funeral mass, and it was exactly what Barbara wanted. As the procession of priest, servers, and attendants started up the aisle, the choir bolted out a revival song with hand clapping and foot stomping. I just smiled a little and looked around the church. It was certainly something different for a Catholic audience used to mild music at a funeral. However, I did notice that I was not the only one with a smile on my face.

Father Charlie was at his best throughout the service. During his homily he had a tough time as he reflected back over Barbara's life. Father Charlie addressed the congregation and said:

"To you Tom, Tommy, and Jason, and to all the family and to all of Barbara's friends, we offer our prayers, our sympathy, and our love. Barbara touched our lives in a wonderful way. She was a real gift to all of us. We were blessed by her presence and her loving touch. On behalf of all the family, I want to thank everyone present here today. Your presence and your prayers mean so much! A special thank you to the choir today from Pentecostal Church who have graced us with their presence. You are a blessing to us all today. Barbara requested no sadness at her funeral, only happy memories, only joyful praise to God because she shares the victory of Jesus. She shares the infinite joy of the Kingdom of God. And your singing lifts our hearts. Thank you. At times like this, it's the presence and care of family and friends that means so much. It's there that we find comfort and support. It's above all, our faith that gives us hope and peace today; our faith that tells us we are beloved of God, and that this world with its joys and sorrows, is not all there is. That death is not the end, only a passage to a far greater life, a life free from disease and pain and all our human limitations. We view death through the eyes of faith."

Father Charlie went on to discuss the importance of faith, love, and the purpose of dying. He concluded the homily by saying, "Barbara, we love you, we will miss you; but we believe in Jesus and his promises. We know that one day we will be reunited." He then read two letters written the night before by my sons. At the end of the mass, Father Charlie said his final prayers as the congregation joined in and commended her soul to Jesus.

After the funeral mass we had a big reception at my parents' house for family and close friends. There was a lot of food, drinks, and conversation among the guests. Most of them did not stay late because of flight times to various locations around the United States the next morning. So the "celebration of life" party that Barbara asked me to have for her was the second on the list of requests that I fulfilled on her behalf.

The next morning I had to say good-bye to my two sons as Tommy returned to his job in Miami, Oklahoma, and Jason went back to the university in Lawrence, Kansas. Tommy told me before he left that he would try to get a transfer to Pennsylvania to be closer to me. I told him that it was a kind thought, but for now he should remain in Oklahoma.

I stayed in Leavenworth for another week, played a lot of golf, and talked to some old friends that still lived in the area. Every day the thought of leaving family and friends to return to a home in Carlisle without my spouse was haunting. But the time had come, and I had to leave.

On my flight back to Harrisburg, I tried to reflect back on all the events that had occurred over the past few months. I knew that I was physically and emotionally exhausted. I needed rest and a new focus on life as I began to deal with the grieving process. I thought a lot about Barbara and all the joy that she had brought into my life. I remembered her beautiful smile and kindness that she shared with everyone. I remembered a conversation that we had in the hospital before she died. She took my hand and thanked me for all that I had done for her. She said, "I am very grateful to God for my life. I have lived a wonderful life and have two wonderful sons. I am grateful that this did not happen to you when the boys were young. At least now they are grown men and you would not have the burden of raising them by yourself." I looked at her and told her that I loved her and appreciated her concern. It was a moment that summarized our life together. She always thought of others before herself.

As my plane began its final decent into Harrisburg International Airport, I had one final thought before I began my new life alone, "No matter what happens to me, I will always reserve a small spot in my heart for the woman I loved and who fought such a courageous battle to beat a deadly disease."

ABOUT THE AUTHOR

✦

THOMAS E. BROWN JR.

AUTHOR OF

Men Bleed Too

Tom was born and raised in Leavenworth, Kansas, and graduated from The University of Kansas in 1970 with a Bachelor of Arts degree. He also holds a Master of Science degree from Emporia State University. In 1992 Tom's first wife, Barbara, was diagnosed with breast cancer. After fighting cancer for nearly two years, Barbara died after a long and courageous struggle. In 1994 Tom met a wonderful woman in Carlisle, Pennsylvania, who also had just lost her spouse to death. Tom and Connie were married on September 30, 1995, and began a new life. Tom and Connie's extended family include three married sons and five grandchildren. Tom retired as a colonel from the United States Army in 1996. After retirement from the service, he and Connie moved to Leavenworth, Kansas, where they now reside. Tom began work on Men Bleed Too *as a journal capturing the events that took place during Barbara's battle with cancer. With Connie's encouragement, he decided to turn the journal into a book.* Men Bleed Too *is a heart-touching story that will affect many lives. In addition to* Men Bleed Too, *Tom is the author of numerous articles published by the U.S. Army. Tom has already started his second book, titled* She Taught Me to Laugh Again. *In this book, Tom relates the story of how he and Connie met, helped each other through the grieving process, and moved forward with their lives. In addition to writing, Tom also works as a consultant for the U.S. Army in computer simulations. Tom is also the co-owner of MarCon, LLC, a properties management business in Leavenworth. His hobbies include woodworking and golf.*

978-0-595-36187-8
0-595-36187-0